JO HARDY

with Caro Handley

Tales from a

Wild Vet

PAWS, CLAWS AND FURRY ENCOUNTERS

HarperElement
An imprint of HarperCollins*Publishers*
1 London Bridge Street
London SE1 9GF

www.harpercollins.co.uk

First published by HarperElement 2016

1 3 5 7 9 10 8 6 4 2

A catalogue record of this book is
available from the British Library

ISBN 978-0-00-814250-6

Printed and bound in Great Britain by
Clays Ltd, St Ives plc

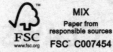

MIX
Paper from
responsible sources
FSC® C007454

CHAPTER ONE

Mickey and the Miracle

'There's something wrong with Mickey. Can you help?'

The elderly couple standing in front of me were visibly upset. She had tears in her eyes, and his lower jaw was trembling.

'He's off his food. He's normally so full of life, but for the last couple of days he's been so quiet. And this morning he was sick and there was ... blood,' they told me.

I looked at the small brown-and-white mutt sitting on the examining table, looking up at me solemnly with big, trusting brown eyes.

'Hello, Mickey,' I said. 'What's up with you then?'

He was a mixed-breed terrier; there was probably a bit of Westie and a bit of Yorkie mixed in with some Cairn in his background. His eyes peered out through a fringe of white hair and his small silky ears flopped over at a perky angle.

I looked at his worried owners. 'Let me take a look at

him while you tell me a bit more about what's been going on. How old is Mickey?'

His owners, Mr and Mrs Thomas, told me that he was seven, which is still fairly young for a small dog. He was a rescue dog, they explained. They'd found him at a dog pound when he was just a puppy and they'd been devoted to him ever since.

As I went through a basic examination, which Mickey tolerated patiently, I rattled through a mental index of possible causes for a dog vomiting blood. The trouble was, it could mean so many things. Had he swallowed a foreign body? Did he have a tumour? Did he have gastritis? Did he have stomach ulcers? Did he have worms? Or might it be an infection?

This was my very first case as a fully qualified vet, and it had to be a complicated one. I had been hoping for something simple; a dose of worms, perhaps, or a vaccination and a bit of flea advice. Instead, here was Mickey, with his mystery condition.

It was early August 2014 and I had been a vet for all of three weeks. After graduating from the Royal Veterinary College (RVC) I'd signed on with an agency as a locum and here I was, on my first day at Braxton's, a small practice in East London, filling in for two weeks while the regular vets were on holiday.

After five long years of study and training, I could still hardly believe that I'd actually made it. We'd been pushed to the limit – and never more so than in our final year, when we'd worked on rotation in every kind of practice, from small animal to stable, to farm and even the zoo. It was non-stop; sometimes terrifying and constantly demanding. But no matter how tough the challenges, there had always been a qualified vet supervising everything I did. Now I suddenly felt as if I'd had the safety net whisked out from under me. For the first time, I was on my own.

I took a deep breath. 'I think we need to give Mickey an X-ray to see what's going on in his stomach. There are a number of things that could be wrong and hopefully that will give us a much better idea of what it is and whether he might need surgery.'

Mickey's owners looked at me, white-faced. 'Will it cost much?' said Mrs Thomas. 'Because we don't have pet insurance and we haven't got a lot of money.'

My heart sank. The sum they mentioned wouldn't cover the X-ray, let alone surgery, which could potentially run into hundreds of pounds. At college they'd taught us to diagnose and treat, but they'd given us very little advice about what to do in financially restricted situations.

In an ideal world, you would want to get a specific diagnosis and treat it directly, but I was becoming increasingly aware that the situation with Mickey was far from ideal. At this stage, Mickey didn't seem like he was critically ill, and it also didn't seem like he had an obstruction, since he was passing stools, so I felt confident that we could trial some treatments and come back to talk about further diagnostics if he didn't improve, maybe with some financial help from a charity. So for now all I could do was give Mickey the medication that his owners could afford and hope it would be enough. I stroked him gently while I attempted a confident smile. 'Don't worry, there are a few things we can do that will hopefully help Mickey.'

I gave him a shot of steroids to bring down the inflammation in his stomach, plus a wormer and a rehydration electrolyte solution to drink and told them not to feed him for 24 hours to allow his stomach to settle, and then to give him a bland diet of boiled rice and chicken.

'Keep a close eye on him,' I said. 'And if he isn't improving in two days, bring him back in.'

'Thank you so much. We will. Come on, Mickey,' they murmured, tucking him into Mrs Thomas's jacket. They left looking a little happier and I crossed my fingers and hoped they wouldn't need to return.

'Fancy a cup of tea?' Karina, the practice nurse, asked.

'Yes, please,' I said gratefully. 'And any chance of a biscuit?'

That morning, at the small hotel where I was staying, I'd been too nervous to eat breakfast. I normally love breakfast, but the prospect of starting my first real job had my stomach doing flips.

I had arrived at the practice bright and early and Karina had greeted me warmly.

'Are any of the regular vets here?' I had asked.

'No.' She smiled. 'All three of them have gone away at the same time. It's just you and another locum.'

I had tried not to look as alarmed as I felt. I had been hoping for a bit of hand-holding as I eased my way in, but there was clearly no chance of that. The other locum, Wanda, came in a couple of minutes later. She was from New Zealand and after we'd said hello she told me she had qualified 18 months earlier. At least she had a bit more experience than I did, but there was no getting round the fact that the place had been left to two vets who were unfamiliar with the practice.

Luckily we had Karina to help us. She was bubbly and smiley and knew her way around, which was a relief, because when we peered around the waiting-room door on that Monday morning we saw that it was already packed with animals and their owners. Karina offered to come into the consulting room with me to help me find my feet and I accepted gratefully. Just having her there, chattering away, made me feel much happier.

'You only get 10 minutes per consultation here,' she had announced cheerfully. I looked at her, feeling daunted. As vet students at the Royal Veterinary College's state-of-the-art Queen Mother Hospital (known as the QMH) we'd had a whole 40 minutes in which to take the animal's history in minute detail and perform the initial examination, before referring our suggested course of treatment to a senior clinician. Most practices allow 15 minutes, but some busy ones across the country have shorter consults, so 10 was going to be high pressure.

At least I had only agreed to do consultations. I didn't feel ready to perform surgery on my own yet, without a more senior vet around. Wanda had agreed to do any surgery that cropped up, and thankfully she seemed fine about it.

After Mickey had disappeared with his owners, he remained on my mind. He was such a sweet little dog, I just hoped that whatever was wrong with him wouldn't turn out to be serious and that the treatments I'd given him would sort out the problem.

The rest of the morning flew by and over a sandwich lunch Wanda and I compared notes. I told her about Mickey and she said she'd been bitten by an angry cat and had to put a very sick hamster to sleep.

Wanda was one of those people with a totally upbeat nature. She spoke with an accent so heavy that I had to concentrate to follow what she was saying. So I wondered if I'd heard her right when she announced that she was off to get a tattoo that night.

'Really?' I said. 'A tattoo? I'd never be able to decide what to have. Plus they really hurt, right?'

'Ah, won't bother me,' Wanda said. 'I'll just put a stick between my teeth and bite hard.' She laughed as she got to her feet. 'Better go, I've got a cat to spay and a pregnant guinea pig to look at.'

After a long afternoon, most of which seemed to be filled with overweight dogs, I began to feel as though the day would never end. When the final patient had left, I said goodnight to Karina and Wanda and gratefully went back to my hotel. Too tired to eat a proper meal, I bought some Pot Noodles on the way and ate them in my room where, thankfully, there was a kettle.

Locum work is tough for a vet straight out of college, but I'd chosen to do it rather than take a full-time job in a practice because I was planning to spend much of the next year travelling. I wanted to see some of the wilder parts of the world and to work in areas where people had no access to a vet.

My first stop would be South Africa in a few months' time, where I was going to work with the SPCA – the Society for the Prevention of Cruelty to Animals.

After a couple of months volunteering with the SPCA I

was planning to fly to Uganda to work for a month with a charity called World in Need, helping villagers in a remote northern area of the country, where there was no vet, to look after their goats, pigs and cows. I would be living miles from the city in a small mud house with no running water or electricity and visiting far-flung homes on foot or by bicycle. I enjoyed my home comforts, so it was definitely going to be a challenge!

I would be back in England for a few more weeks of work after that, before heading off on another adventure, this time to Morocco to work with a charity caring for injured horses and donkeys.

With all that to come I felt both excited and nervous. But, meanwhile, I needed to get a bit of experience under my belt, and earn some money.

On my third morning at Braxton's the sun was out, the birds were chirping as I walked to work and I felt sure the day was going to be a good one.

In reception I found Wanda and Karina waiting for the kettle to boil and laughing.

'Morning!' I said. 'What's the joke?'

'This,' Wanda said, pulling up her sleeve to reveal a tattoo that covered her entire arm.

I gasped. 'Wow! When you said you were getting a tattoo I didn't think you meant ...'

'Ha!' laughed Wanda. 'You thought I was going to go for some neat little bluebird tucked away by my shoulder? Nope, this is what's known as a full-sleeve. And when it's settled down,' she regarded her swollen arm, with its crust of dried blood, 'it's going to look just beaut.'

'I bet it is,' I replied. 'What's the picture, exactly? It's hard to tell.'

'That,' Wanda said proudly, 'is known as The Tribal. It's based on tribal Maori designs. Did I tell you I've got a bit of Maori heritage? This is my way of celebrating it.'

I had to laugh. Wanda was completely nuts but it was impossible not to like her.

The morning passed peacefully with a few routine cases and I felt I was just getting into my stride when Mr and Mrs Thomas appeared with a very subdued-looking Mickey. He hadn't perked up at all. In fact, the poor little thing looked much worse.

He lay flat out on the examining table, showing no interest in anything at all. Mrs Thomas, her eyes red-rimmed, told me he hadn't wanted to eat anything at all. He had stopped vomiting, but that was probably because he hadn't eaten, as clearly he wasn't on the mend.

I felt so sorry for him, and for the Thomases. He was their world and they were terrified of losing him. I promised I would give him anything I had that might possibly help.

I started with anti-emetics to help with his nausea and vomiting, gastro-protectants to help with any inflammation in his gastro-intestinal tract, and antibiotics in case he had a bacterial infection. As I watched his very downcast owners take him home again, I could only hope that one or all of these drugs would do the trick.

But the following day Mickey and his owners were back.

'Nothing seems to be working,' Mrs Thomas told me as she brought Mickey out from inside her jacket.

The little chap was weak and could barely lift his head. Something was clearly very wrong and I was running out of options.

I looked at Mr and Mrs Thomas, both of whom were on the verge of tears. 'I think I'd better keep him here overnight,' I said. 'He's dehydrated because he's not eating or drinking much. I can put him on a drip and give him intravenous fluids and that should help.'

They agreed and, shoulders bowed, they left their precious little dog with me. I carried Mickey gently through to the little hospital room in the back and set him up on a drip. I tried to feed him some high-calorie paste from my finger. He ignored it, so I heated it up a little to make it warm and slightly smellier. He showed some mild interest and while he licked at it half-heartedly, I stroked him. 'Come on, Mickey, you can do it. Please don't give up,' I whispered.

I checked on him every hour or so and that night he seemed settled. Wanda, who was staying in the flat over the surgery, promised to come down and check on him again before she went to bed.

That night I talked to my boyfriend, Jacques, on Skype. He was 6,000 miles away in South Africa and I missed him. He listened patiently to all my tales of woe and did his best to cheer me up when I told him about Mickey, but it wasn't the same as having him there with me. I could have done with one of his warm hugs.

After a sleepless night I arrived at work early the next morning. Much to my delight, Mickey had picked up a little, so I phoned the Thomases and suggested they come and get him and carry on nursing him at home. They were delighted to find him a little brighter and they took him home, along with some of the high-calorie paste. The following day, though, Mrs Thomas rang to say that Mickey was still very ill.

It was Friday. I had thrown every treatment that they could afford at him. I explained to Mrs Thomas that of course it was up to her and her husband to decide what to do, but that if Mickey didn't improve over the weekend it might mean that he wasn't going to get better.

'Does that mean we should have him put to sleep?' Mrs Thomas asked, her voice shaky.

'Well, we don't want him to suffer, so in the end it might be the kindest thing,' I answered.

That night I went back to my family home in Tunbridge Wells for the weekend. My parents had lived in the same house since I was a year old and it was always good to go home and see them and our dogs: springer spaniel Tosca, and Yorkshire terrier Paddy.

On Saturday I spent time with my horses, Elli and Tammy, riding and grooming them. I'd had horses ever since I was a little girl and I adored them. It was a beautiful summer weekend, the kind you seldom get in an English August, but Mickey was constantly in my thoughts. I knew his owners would be heartbroken if I had to put him to sleep and I wished there was something more I could do for him.

Monday morning arrived and I was back in East London. Mickey was booked in as the last of my consultations that day, and I was dreading it; I hate putting animals to sleep, although I'm always glad to be able to relieve suffering. But when I went out to the waiting room, much to my surprise, there, sitting between his owners, was a decidedly perkier Mickey. And what's more, Mr and Mrs Thomas both had great big grins on their faces.

In the consulting room they explained that they'd brought Mickey in to show me how much he had improved – and I could see that he had. Relief flooded through me and I thanked goodness that the treatment had worked. As I stroked the rough fur on his small head it took all my willpower to stop myself from shedding a tear.

'I'm so glad the treatment worked!' I said.

Mrs Thomas patted my hand.

'Oh no, dear, it wasn't you,' she said. 'On Sunday one of our friends prayed for Mickey and he started to brighten up right away. It was a miracle.'

I said nothing and smiled. I was just delighted that he was looking so much better. In the end, did it really matter whether it was down to my treatments or a bit of divine intervention?

CHAPTER TWO

Hedgehogs, Doves and a Very Cross Pheasant

Two beady eyes regarded me intently from a bed of straw inside the cardboard box, and a small, pointed snout twitched curiously.

'Can you help?' the little girl asked over the top of the reception desk at Folly Wildlife Rescue, where I was volunteering. 'It came out of the bonfire Dad lit in the garden. We didn't know it was in there, we're so sorry.' Her eyes filled with tears.

'We'll do our best,' I said. 'Let me take him from you and we'll have a look.'

Very carefully I lifted the hedgehog out of the box and onto the table. Some spines were missing on his back and there was a nasty wound on his side, clearly a burn. Heather, one of the animal care assistants at the centre, got to work cleaning the wound with antiseptic.

'I don't think he's going to die, but we need to treat him and keep him here for a little while. The spines he's lost won't grow back – they can't grow through scar tissue – but he can survive without them and the wound should heal. Give us a call in a few weeks and if he's recovered you can take him home and release him back into your garden.'

The little girl – she couldn't have been more than eight – wiped away her tears and smiled. 'Really? Can we come back, Daddy?' She turned to her father, who was standing behind her.

'Of course,' he said. 'We'll come and see how he's doing, and when he's ready we'll take him back and let him go. And next time I light a fire at the bottom of the garden I'll check first.'

As father and daughter left, hand in hand, after generously giving a small donation to the charity, I took the hedgehog through to where an empty cage was waiting for him and laid him gently inside. I had applied antibiotic cream to his wound and would keep a close eye on him to make sure he was healing. I filled in the chart on the front of his cage and a few moments later, Julie, one of the volunteers, came through with a little dish of scrambled eggs.

'Here's a treat for him. This should perk him up a bit.'

In between locum jobs I was spending several mornings working as a volunteer at a rescue charity for injured and orphaned wild animals. Folly Wildlife Rescue is an amazing place, home to dozens of hedgehogs, as well as badgers, foxes, deer, ducks and birds. Most of them are brought in by members of the public, and once they arrive at Folly the animals are treated, fed and cared for until they have recovered enough to be released into the wild again.

Open 24 hours a day, Folly was first set up by husband-and-wife team Dave and Annette Risley. It started in their back garden, with sheds, aviaries and hutches, and bit by bit they raised the funds to build the fantastic well-equipped centre they have now.

When you arrive at Folly, in Broadwater Forest, not far from where I live in Tunbridge Wells, you're greeted with a cacophony of cooing and chirping, because the wall beside the reception desk is stacked with birdcages three or four tiers high.

Go past reception and you find yourself in the Intensive Care Unit (ICU). Here you will be greeted by two tiers of incubators for younger birds or small mammals or for the older ones that need intensive care, alongside a whole wall of bigger cages for recovering birds and small furries, plus a large examination table in the middle for checking over all the newly admitted animals. Beyond the ICU is the hedgehog ward: dozens of white, glass-fronted, ventilated cages – all of them full – alongside work surfaces for feeding, weighing and examining the animals daily.

Finally there is the 'other animals' ward, where badgers,

rabbits, pheasants and the odd stoat, owl or duck reside. This ward has bigger cages and two small rooms attached to it where the larger animals can move around a bit better. The charity has a second site for rescued deer and there is another local charity that deals with foxes, so these animals are rarely seen in this hospital.

In all the wards every cage door has a chart attached to it, with details of when the animal arrived, its weight, diagnosis and the treatment and food it's being given.

I first worked at Folly when I started my vet training, when I did a week's work experience. Back then I helped to clean cages and feed the animals, but now that I was a qualified vet I was put to work examining and diagnosing the new arrivals and helping to decide on and administer treatment.

The centre is staffed by three well-trained, resourceful animal care assistants, alongside Annette and Dave and several willing volunteers, but there was no vet. They were trying to raise funds at the time to build a fully equipped vet suite, which I was only too happy to advise Dave on, with the intention of eventually employing a full-time vet. In the meantime, though, they were glad of any passing vet who was happy to come in and help out.

The little hedgehog caught in the bonfire is typical of the patients that people bring in to centres like Folly. It is sadly all too common for hedgehogs, which live in close proximity to humans, to be caught in bonfires, attacked by dogs, run over by lawnmowers (or cars), or to slip into garden ponds or be trapped in fencing. Sometimes they're found wandering about during the day when they should be sleeping. That usually means they're short of food. Sometimes they are found sick – with mange, lungworm or mites – or simply struggling to survive because they've been born too late in the year and haven't put on enough weight to be able to hibernate and survive their first winter.

Hedgehogs are Britain's favourite wild creature. Immortalised in Beatrix Potter's much-loved story of Mrs Tiggy-Winkle, as well as in numerous books and poems by literary giants such as the poet Philip Larkin, everyone loves them. Yet sadly they're becoming a rare sight and are even at risk of becoming endangered. Over the past 50 years it is estimated that hedgehog numbers have fallen from around 36 million in the UK to fewer than a million, largely due to loss of their natural habitat. With fewer wilderness areas, hedgehogs are short of both food and safe spaces in which to live and nest. Thousands of them die on the roads, and while looking for food they often stray into gardens that can be full of dangers to them.

There are 17 species of hedgehog; little mammals whose spines are made of hollow hairs hardened by keratin, the stuff that human hair and nails are made from. A distant relative of the shrew (but nothing to do with porcupines), hedgehogs are believed to have changed very little in the past 15 million years, so it would be heartbreaking if we lost them now.

Folly is one of the places doing their utmost to save hedgehogs, by nursing back to health those injured animals that are brought in and by raising awareness of these little creatures and their habits and habitats. If everyone kept a little bit of wilderness in the corner of a garden, made sure that the animals could get out of the garden through a hole in the fence, and looked out for hedgehogs when building ponds or fires, it would make a real difference to their survival rate.

My next case there that day was a mother hedgehog and her two tiny babies, all of them riddled with mites. Their skin was raw and itchy and they'd lost quite a few spines. Mite infestation is very common in hedgehogs; the mites are parasites that are usually too small to see, but they're easy to treat with the same spot treatment you use for dogs.

Before we applied the spot-on treatment (to avoid it getting washed off) we gave them a family bath in a washing-up bowl containing an inch of warm water with baby oil in it, to soothe their skin and keep it nice and soft.

They loved it and we soon had them settled comfortably in a cage together, tucking into a bowl of cat food. Hedgehogs love cat or dog food, scrambled eggs and, as a special treat, rusks soaked in goat's milk, as they are unable to digest cows' milk properly. All of these treats are prepared in the centre's kitchen, which is just along from the 'other animals' ward. Making up a load of delicious food, all served on plant-pot saucers, was a lot of fun. I enjoyed being chef to 30 little creatures!

The hedgehogs were easy to work with, too, as long as you managed to avoid the spines and didn't mind the vast amount of faeces that came out of them, no matter how much or how little they ate. The birds, on the other hand, well, they could be a bit of a challenge, especially the collared doves. And there were a lot of collared doves.

Pigeons and doves are very similar; they all belong to the bird family Columbidae, though traditionally the name dove tends to be used for the smaller species and pigeon for the larger ones. I hadn't had a lot of experience of working with birds before I went to Folly, but during my time there I learned a lot more about them and it really helped my confidence in interacting with them. I hadn't ever thought much of pigeons, but since being around lots of them I have discovered that they're friendly, silly birds that you can't help liking.

Even more surprising is that the different varieties have very different personalities. The collared doves are notoriously naughty and not very bright. They're like thoroughbred horses: no brains and lots of energy. The second you opened their cages they would shoot out, which made it extremely hard to treat them. Each time one of them escaped the receptionist would yell, 'Windows!' and we'd all race to shut every window and door to stop the bird getting out. Then we'd face the tricky job of recapturing it, which usually took at least 10 minutes and often required the use of a net, which stood propped up in the corner ready for this all-too-common scenario.

When they weren't escaping the collared doves were trying to peck you. I had to handle one with a swollen eye – it had a virus known as pox and it needed eye drops. Many of the other birds needed oral medication and, after a few unsuccessful attempts, thanks to Heather I learned a good way of holding the head so that the bird couldn't move or peck me. I put two fingers on either side of the beak and two fingers behind the head. Not only did it keep them still, it allowed me to open the beak so that I could pop medicine in for the ones that needed oral medication or to feed those that weren't eating properly.

The wood pigeons were a whole lot easier. Their main concern was food, so far from trying to escape they would settle in happily for the free feeds. They'd quickly get the idea that we would hand-feed them when they were sick, and started begging like dogs, especially the younger ones, jumping up and down at the front of the cage, making a squawking racket. Then, when you took them out, they would happily open their mouths wide ready for food.

While some breeds of pigeon were common at Folly, a racing pigeon was a rare sight, so when one was brought in one morning we all crowded round to have a look. Larger and far more slender than the other pigeons, this bird looked like pigeon royalty. There was nothing wrong with him, apart from the fact that he had got lost and a member of the public had caught him and brought him in, thinking he must belong to someone since he had a ring on his leg. The ID on the ring was bringing up no results, which was perhaps a good thing; pigeon racing is a competitive sport and many racers don't have the space to keep pigeons that get lost or aren't fit enough to complete the distance, so if his owner had been traced the fate of the pigeon might have been quite uncertain. Instead, the pigeon was boarded while we waited to see if an owner would come forward. If not, the ring would be removed and the pigeon would either be allowed to live out his days in the large aviaries on site, which are for birds that cannot be rereleased, or rehomed.

Many of the wild pigeons brought in to Folly were suffering from canker, or trichomonas. It's a horrible disease in which white clots build up in the bird's throat that prevent it from swallowing or breathing properly. Eighty per cent of pigeons carry the organism, but they don't all become infected. When the birds become stressed the organism can multiply and a mild infection can turn into a serious condition.

Pigeons with canker have to be given antibiotics and need to be crop-fed, which means their food has to be pushed past the clots and into the bird's crop, which is the muscular pouch near the gullet or throat. The crop is basically an expanded part of the oesophagus and it's used to temporarily store food.

Learning to crop-feed was another bird-handling skill I acquired at Folly. The receptionist, Poppy, an elderly lady of great character, was particularly helpful with this one.

'When the crop feels like a scrotum you've got the food in properly,' she said breezily.

'A-ha, thanks,' I said, laughing so hard I almost dropped the tube of mashed Weetabix mixed with recovery formula that I was using to feed a small wood pigeon.

But not all birds needed hand-feeding, many could feed themselves on bird seed, depending on their age and the severity of their injury or disease.

Birds would often come in with injuries after being mauled by cats. One family arrived with a baby collared dove that had puncture wounds all over its back. The poor little thing was traumatised. We cleaned the wounds and treated them with antibiotics, and as we did so I learned a useful tip from the animal care assistants at Folly; they would take an antibiotic capsule meant for swallowing, open it up and sprinkle the powder on the bird's wounds. It was an unconventional method, but it worked extremely well.

Like the hedgehogs, the pigeons are rehabilitated and released back into the wild whenever possible. The members of the public who bring them in the first place are usually happy to take them back and release them in the place where they were found, which is the best approach for the animals.

The pigeons were hard work, but the biggest challenge I faced at Folly was in fact a large male pheasant. He was big and strong and he did not like being in captivity. He had an injured leg – a healing fracture – and he needed pain relief and rest, but every time I opened his cage to give him his medication and check on his leg, or give his cage a bit of a clean, he made a break for it. In that moment, he always forgot about his painful leg – escape was the only thing on his mind. He was so strong and flapped his wings so hard that it was difficult to get near him; even when I did catch him with my hands, he was so strong and powerful that he regularly managed to break away, so I ended up having to herd him back into his cage, shooing and clapping behind him while the other workers cut off all available exits.

The pheasant was not happy, but after several weeks at Folly his leg had healed and he was ready for release. Folly is situated in a beautiful forest, so it was decided that he could be released into a new habitat, away from roads or any areas in which pheasant hunting is common. I was given the privilege of letting him go, so after battling to get him into a cat carrier, I walked him down the driveway. He was not impressed. I felt him battering the box from the inside, but when I got to the edge of the wood I set the box on the ground and opened the door. Sprinting out, flapping his wings, he took flight for 10 metres or so, before hitting the ground and disappearing at top speed into the darkness of the wood. Watching him fly away was a wonderful feeling.

Folly is an amazing resource; I loved volunteering there and have gone back since to take them a baby sparrow that had fallen out of its nest at the stables where my horses are kept. The little thing had hit its head, which was swollen, but with a bit of Folly's tender and expert care it recovered and, too young to be released, stayed to be hand-reared at the centre until it was big enough to fend for and feed itself.

One afternoon, after a morning at Folly, I set off to visit my friend Lucy, who was living in a small village in West Sussex. Lucy and I had met at the RVC in our third year and in our final year we'd been in the same rotation group of five students, sharing all our core placements.

We'd been close friends ever since. Lucy is an amazing person; a brilliant and talented vet as well as clever and forthright and a lot of fun. It was Lucy who kept me sane during the toughest moments of our training, and Lucy who commiserated with me when things went wrong.

After we graduated Lucy had headed straight for farm work, winning a highly sought-after internship with a small farm-based veterinary practice that would, hopefully, lead to a permanent job. She was only an hour away from my family's home, so we'd promised to meet up often, but in the weeks since graduation we'd both been so busy that three months had gone by before we could find a time to get together. I was longing to see her and looking forward to catching up.

Lucy was living in a pretty little terraced house with a cottagey feel to it that she shared with another vet and the black cocker spaniel she had bought soon after we graduated. She'd called him Renly, after her favourite character in *Game of Thrones*, and he was gorgeous and cuddly but very, very naughty. He had just been castrated and Lucy said she was feeling very sorry for him, but he didn't appear to be suffering – he was leaping everywhere and making inroads into the kitchen bin every time Lucy turned her back, so that the house rang with constant cries of, 'Renly, no!'

Over a delicious dinner and a glass of wine, Lucy told me all about her new life. She had settled into the practice and was becoming part of the farm community and I could see how much she was enjoying it. She said she was working hard, going from farm to farm with Renly tucked into a crate in the back of her car, but the work was what she had always enjoyed most, and she was being given lots of support by the vets in the practice.

Lucy was full of stories about her work. One of the funniest was about a pig called Patsy that appeared to be so ill it couldn't stand up. Lucy arrived at the farm with a vet student in tow and examined the pig, taking its temperature with a thermometer up its backside. It was clearly unwell and she suspected pneumonia, but when she went to inject it with antibiotics and anti-inflammatories the pig, which weighed all of 200 kilos, suddenly leaped to its feet, the needle still stuck in its rump, and shot straight into a bush from which it refused to emerge. Clearly after the indignity of the thermometer, the injection was a step too far. After failing to chase the pig out, Lucy and the vet student stood in the field trying to tempt it out with apples and bran mash, at which point Lucy finally managed to retrieve her syringe and make a hasty exit.

It was lovely to spend an evening with Lucy; she made me laugh, gave me a great meal and reminded me of how precious good friends are. I was so pleased for her that she had settled into country life, but I couldn't help thinking how different our lives were now, with Lucy in a stable job with a house and a dog, while the next year for me was going to be filled with travelling, both in the UK and abroad.

In the end, though, I decided that both options were exciting, just in different ways.

CHAPTER THREE

Tosca

Mine is a family of animal-lovers. In particular, dogs. We've always had dogs, mostly springer spaniels; affectionate, loyal and energetic companions. Tosca had been part of our family since I was 11. I could barely remember a time when she hadn't been around. Whenever I had gone home from veterinary college she was waiting to leap up at me, pawing at me when I ignored her and demanding my instant and undivided attention.

A pretty black-and-white springer spaniel, you always knew when Tosca was around. If you tried to sit down with a book she'd nudge your hand with one of her beloved tennis balls, inviting you to go and throw it for her, then bounding around in delight when you gave in to her demands, put your book down and went outside with her. You'd throw it and she'd run after it, but instead of bringing it back she'd start playing with it, and then dig a hole to bury it. She never did get the hang of retrieving. After every meal Tosca would lick all the plates as we loaded them into the dishwasher, hovering ready to snap up any scrap that was inadvertently dropped and oblivious to exasperated groans of, 'No, Tosca, leave it alone.' She was the undisputed definition of naughty.

Ironically, Tosca didn't like me when she first arrived as a puppy; she seemed to see me as her rival in the pecking order (Ross, my younger brother, on the other hand, she dismissed as bottom!). She would growl at me, and I would snarl back, until we both thought we had won. But our relationship grew from this unpromising beginning into something deep and unique. I used to love curling up on the sofa with her, stroking her soft, floppy ears as she rested her head on my lap. When I was studying for exams – first GCSEs, then A levels, then the endless exams through five years of vet school – Tosca always seemed to know. She'd suddenly suspend her usual demands and come and sit quietly beside me, as if she understood that I needed her support. So when, at the beginning of my fourth year at vet school, Tosca became ill and almost died, I was devastated.

By the time I left home for college we'd had Tosca for over eight years and our little Yorkshire terrier, Paddy, for four. Paddy was only eight months old when we got him and was just a little brown ball of fur. He'd been rescued from a house in which around 200 Yorkshire terriers had been found after their elderly owner died; some of them dead, the rest suffering from disease and malnutrition. Paddy had escaped relatively unscathed and he and Tosca soon bonded – she took him under her wing and they'd snuggle on the sofa together.

Then one Saturday, when I was home from college for the weekend, I found Tosca lying on her side groaning, her belly horribly swollen. She had gorged herself on the sack of dried dog food we kept hidden away in the conservatory. We couldn't think what was going on, or even how she'd got to it – Tosca was a bit of a scavenger, but she'd never done that before. In recent weeks, though, she'd had other episodes of behaving oddly, such as hiding in strange places so that we had to hunt for her.

She had drunk a lot of water after eating the food, which had made it swell in her stomach. We took her to Louise, our local out-of-hours vet, who decided that Tosca would need surgery, as there was too much in her stomach for it to be eliminated naturally.

Louise operated that evening, but when I phoned to see how Tosca was doing, Louise told me she wasn't coming round from the anaesthetic as easily as she should. When Tosca finally did wake up she was in a bad way – her condition was critical. And as the life of my dear, faithful exam-buddy hung in the balance, I had to return to college after the weekend and anxiously await updates from home.

The following day, Mum phoned. Tosca had been referred as an emergency to the Queen Mother Hospital, which was attached to the Royal Veterinary College where I was studying. My parents were on their way right now with Tosca in their car, as it was quicker than waiting for a pet ambulance. I waited outside the hospital until they swung into the car park. When I opened the boot I was shocked to see that our lovely energetic and bouncy dog couldn't even stand up. She was attached to a drip and was limp and lifeless.

Inside the hospital she was whisked away by vets and nurses and a little while later the senior clinician, Giacomo, called us in to explain that Tosca's abdomen had become septic after her operation and as a consequence her heart had started beating in an irregular rhythm that could be fatal. Even with further surgery to flush out the infected fluid and medication for her heart, she would only have a 50/50 chance of survival.

We were stunned. Tosca couldn't die; we weren't ready to lose her. We were allowed to go through and give her a cuddle before she was taken into surgery. After several hours of anxious waiting I was told that she had made it through the operation but was still in a critical condition. In addition to her stomach problems they had found a small tumour on her adrenal gland. Once again she hadn't come round as expected, which the vets felt might indicate that she also had a brain tumour which was causing the anaesthetic to be filtered out of her brain more slowly than usual.

The news that she had cancer as well as septic peritonitis was pretty devastating, but there was still hope. The cancer was in the early stages and could be a slow-growing type, so there was a good chance that, if she made it through this ordeal, she would have another couple of years.

Tosca remained in the Intensive Care Unit for three weeks. It was a tough time for all of us, but with the expert care of the vets and nurses, she pulled through. As a vet student I was allowed to visit her often and I spent a lot of time in her kennel, talking to her, cuddling her and sitting beside her with my textbooks open on my lap. She had grown painfully thin, but I coaxed her into eating again by gently feeding her sausages, and when she was finally well enough to go home she tottered out of the hospital. All the way home she squealed in the way she did when she wanted a walk, so we knew we had our Tosca back and promised never to complain about her annoying traits again.

We were all thrilled to have her home, and once she was back in her own territory she carried on getting better and soon seemed like her old self. But as the months passed we realised she was losing her sight, and her head had begun to tilt to one side, which meant that she probably did have a slow-growing brain tumour. This may have accounted for the uncharacteristic behaviour that she continued to display, such as hiding in strange places and her gorging episode.

Tosca didn't appear to be too fazed by losing her sight. She still charged around the house, so we put bubble wrap around the trees in the garden and horse boots on the legs of the dining-room chairs so that she wouldn't hurt herself when she bumped into them. She never seemed to have a problem finding us – or the dishwasher – and she still demanded our undivided attention.

When I graduated a year later she was still doing well and we were hopeful that she would be with us for some time yet. After my graduation ceremony and the ball that followed and once all the excitement was over, Jacques and I drove down to Cornwall to join my parents and Ross for a holiday. Every year Mum, Dad, Ross and I go to the same little cottage in the Camel Valley Vineyard in north Cornwall for a lazy fortnight of pottering around beaches, walking the dogs, looking at holiday cottages and filling up with cream teas at Viv's café down the road. This year, Jacques was joining us, and I was looking forward to spending time with him in one of my favourite parts of the country. Jacques and I planned to arrive a few days after the rest of my family, as I had to pack up my house at university and say a sad goodbye to my housemates and friends.

After the long drive from Kent to Cornwall, never less than six hours, Jacques and I pulled up at the vineyard, got out of the car to stretch our aching limbs and lifted our bags out of the boot. We walked down the path towards our cottage to find Mum outside with Tosca lying on the ground beside her in the shade.

I ran towards them. 'What happened?'

'Tosca's been really off colour today,' Mum said. 'We knew you were on the way, so we decided to wait and see what you thought before getting help. Especially as it's Sunday.'

I knelt down and stroked Tosca. She barely responded. Her little tail, seldom still, didn't even manage a small welcoming wag. There was also a faint rattle coming from her chest as she breathed.

'She was playing in the sea yesterday,' Mum said. 'You know how much she loves dashing in and out of the waves. But she can't see them coming and I think she's inhaled some salt water.'

I looked up at Mum. 'She really looks awful. We need to get her to a vet. I can't help her, I have nothing with me.'

We got Tosca gently into the car and took her to a very friendly local out-of-hours vet called Sandra, who took her temperature — which was alarmingly high — gave her an antibiotic injection and a Metacam injection to bring her temperature down and asked us to bring her back in the morning.

A diagnosis was difficult. Given that we knew she had cancer, there might well have been tumours in her lungs. But it was also possible that, having inhaled seawater, she had developed pneumonia.

We took her back to the cottage to rest. The vet told us to make sure she was eating and drinking, but we couldn't persuade her to take anything at all. No small titbit tempted her, not even sausage; she wouldn't even drink water, so the next morning we took her back and she was put on a drip for 24 hours to rehydrate her.

That helped, but when we took her home again she was still very weak. At worst she simply lay flat; at best she managed a small wag of her tail. We took it in turns to check on her and sit with her. None of us wanted to say it, but we were very afraid that we were losing her.

The following day Dad suggested we take her to the beach. It was her favourite place and Dad reasoned that we would either be taking her for one last visit, if she really was reaching the end, or it would give her a boost and she just might perk up. It was kill or cure time.

We all agreed it was a good idea, and once again we lifted her gently into the car before heading down the road to the sea. When we arrived Jacques carried her from the car to the beach where – to all of our delight and amazement – she lifted her head, sniffed the salt air and immediately launched into a shaky jog towards the sea.

We stood, grinning. It was clear that, weak as she was, she was back with us and ready to fight. I hugged Jacques. 'She's tough as old boots,' I said, wiping away a tear. 'She's not ready to go yet.'

'You're right, she's some dog,' he said, watching her with a look of slight incredulity on his face.

After that Tosca gradually regained some of her energy and vitality. She was still weak, but we could all see that her spirit was undimmed. We took her to the beach every day, where she dug a huge number of holes in the sand and continually tried to scamper off towards the sea, bumping into people on the beach that she couldn't see.

At the end of the week Jacques had to go back to South Africa. I drove him to Heathrow where for once I didn't dissolve into tears because I knew that we were only facing a short parting this time; I was going to be joining him for two weeks at the end of August, only a month away.

After seeing Jacques off, I drove to Kent to collect Mum's parents, Grandma and Grandpa Nevison, who lived next door to us. I'm lucky in having my grandparents so close by. Dad's parents, Grandma and Grandpa Hardy, only live half an hour from us, so I've got all four around me and they're all absolutely lovely.

Our second holiday week was deliciously peaceful. Tosca was doing well, the sun shone and we enjoyed long walks and plenty of cream teas. I also managed to pop over to visit my old friend Tom, who runs a dairy farm close to where we were staying. A few years older than me, Tom is a quiet country farmer who took over the farm from his parents. Happy to stay settled in one place, Tom loves his farm, his animals and meeting his friends for a pint down at the pub in the evenings. We are very different, but we get on well. We've known each other for almost 10 years, ever since I spent a few weeks doing work experience on the farm when I was 16, and it's always good to catch up.

Tom asked me to give him a hand with diagnosing his cows' pregnancy, as he had a few he wasn't sure about. Tom had a really old-school diagnosis method called 'ballotte-ment of the abdomen', which is seldom used nowadays because it's so inaccurate. It consists of pushing your hand against the side of the cow and wobbling the tummy around to see if you come up against something – like a calf. The trouble is, it only really works if the foetus is big enough, so the cow has to be at least halfway through a pregnancy for you to be able to pick up her condition.

There was one cow in particular that Tom was very fond of, a pretty black-and-white Holstein. She produced excellent milk yields and had had several calves in the previous few years, but for some reason she hadn't become pregnant for quite a while. With dairy farming these days you can't afford to lose any time. There is a voluntary waiting period of about 40 to 60 days after a cow gives birth when you give her a rest. After that you put her with the bull again, or artificially inseminate her, in the hope that she will fall pregnant within two reproductive cycles of 21 days each. If a cow is not pregnant six months or so after a birth then she becomes expensive to maintain and it's time to think about slaughter or selling on at market.

Tom thought he felt something bumping against his hand and was hoping that this particular cow was pregnant. I checked her rectally, a technique I had had plenty of practice with thanks to my old friend Thys, an eccentric Afrikaner vet I had worked with on my frequent trips to

South Africa while I was training. Thys had taught me always to insert my left hand into the cow, so that I could properly feel the uterus from inside.

'Clarrie's been one of my best cows,' he said, 'and I think I felt something when I checked her, so I'm hoping she's in the family way again now.'

'Clarrie?' I said, eyebrows raised.

Tom looked sheepish. 'I know it's not the wisest thing to do to name them, but she's a lovely cow, and she reminds me of Clarrie in *The Archers* – long-suffering and good-hearted.'

I laughed. 'OK, Tom, let's hope Clarrie is going to make you a happy dad again.'

I inserted my arm and felt her uterus. There was nothing there.

'I'm so sorry, Tom, she's not pregnant.'

His face fell. 'Really? I could have sworn she was. Could you be wrong?'

I turned to him and said, 'Well, I know I'm still freshly graduated, but I'm certain I can't feel anything.'

His face fell. 'I don't believe you.'

'I'll give it a second go, just to make sure,' I said.

Clarrie was none too happy by this time. She'd had enough of my arm up her rump and was trying to shake me off.

'Hang onto her, will you, Tom? She's getting frisky and I'd rather not be trampled on my first outing as a fully-fledged vet, thanks.'

After a second check I pulled off my gloves and turned to Tom.

'I promise you, there's no obvious foetus in there, Tom, unless she's in the early stages, which I can't tell without a scanner. Could that be possible?'

'No, she should be well on by now. Let me feel.' He inserted his hand into the cow. He wasn't happy. 'Oh, Jo, what a shame. This girl is one of my best yielders.'

His shoulders drooped. He knew it was time to send Clarrie to market. For Tom, as for all dairy farmers, with milk prices at an all-time low, hard-headed decisions had to be made.

He looked at me, his expression defiant.

'I know I should let her go,' he said. 'But I'm not going to. Not yet. Clarrie has more than earned her keep until now. I'm going to put her out to pasture and give her a bit longer. She may fall pregnant next time round. She deserves another chance.'

I hesitated. He was making the decision with his heart, not his head. But sometimes we all need to do that.

I smiled. 'OK, Tom, good call. Let's hope she's in calf again in a few months.'

He smiled, relieved. 'Come on then, I think you've earned a slice of Mum's apple pie.'

The following day my phone rang. It was one of the publicity crew from ITN Productions, asking whether I would be willing to do a few interviews to publicise *Young Vets*. This was a television series that had been made in my last year at vet college and it was about to air. Along with nine other student vets from my academic year at the Royal Veterinary College, I had been followed around on most of my work placements by a camera crew. Nerve-wracking at first (who wants to have their mistakes filmed?), within a couple of weeks the crew and I became friends and I barely noticed the cameras. In fact, it felt a bit odd, and even lonely, when they weren't trailing me through every muddy farmyard, stable, operating suite and consulting room. When the series was completed the final shots were of our graduation, the 10 of us leaping in the air with joy.

I said I would be happy to give interviews. We'd been warned that this would be a necessary part of the process when we had first signed up for the series, but I couldn't help feeling horribly nervous. What if I said the wrong thing? What if I made a fool of myself? Or I embarrassed vets everywhere with my comments?

Most of my interviews could be done over the phone, thankfully. At least that way the interviewers wouldn't be able to see how nervous I was, and ITN could supply photos from a shoot we'd done with them. But I still felt distinctly jittery.

After our return from Cornwall it was hard to say goodbye to the family, and especially hard to say goodbye to Tosca, who was still not quite her old self. But that was when I had to go and start my first two weeks of locum work at Braxton's so, waving goodbye to the family, I packed my things into my little car and off I went.

When I got back home after that first stint of locum work I felt absolutely exhausted. It was so good to be home. Mum was cooking a roast chicken for dinner, Dad gave me a big hug and I sat down on the sofa and burst into tears. I was looking forward to a couple of weeks at home now, volunteering at Folly Wildlife Hospital, before heading off for two weeks in the South African sunshine with Jacques – I couldn't wait.

Tosca was still doing well. She was a little more frail than before, but she was still bouncing around and was happy to curl up beside me as I checked the statistics for my research project. During our final year at the RVC we'd all had to carry out a piece of original research; mine was on horses' hooves, and whether wearing horse shoes was ultimately of benefit or if horses were actually better off without them. I'd had to photograph and measure the hooves of a lot of horses and I had put a huge amount of work into it, so I was delighted when my supervisor said he thought that what I'd produced was good enough to be published in a scientific journal. But before I submitted it I had to repeat the measurements to verify that my results – which came down in favour of horses not wearing shoes – were valid and reliable. So I had to painstakingly work through it all again.

Soon after I got home I had a visit from our local ITV news programme, *South East Today*. *Young Vets* was due to air in a couple of days and they wanted an interview. No sooner had I said yes than they confirmed a date and arrived, cameras in tow. We did an interview in the sitting room and then rushed off to the stables so they could show me with my two horses, Elli and Tammy. As they were leaving they said it would be on the lunchtime news that day. That was in two hours' time.

At five to one I turned on the TV and sat down, a plate of cheese toast on my knee, to watch. I hadn't seen the films of *Young Vets* and I still couldn't imagine what it was going to be like watching myself on TV. It was a strange experience. I think it's almost impossible to see yourself on film and not feel critical (why didn't I tuck that lock of hair behind my ear and why do I sound so cheesy?), but it could have been worse.

The news clip was a taste of what was to come. Two days later the whole family sat down to watch the first episode in the *Young Vets* series. I only appeared in the introduction to the first one – I wasn't given a solo slot until Episode Four – so I was able to enjoy watching the others. I grinned at Charlie, one of the friendliest and kindest people I knew, and then Grace, who could appear a bit ditzy but was ultimately an excellent vet.

As soon as the programme got underway the tweets began. I never did get used to reading Twitter comments from people who didn't know me, but when the four episodes in which I had solo sections were aired, there were plenty of them to read. Only one was genuinely unkind and I realised I had been lucky – I could have been mauled. Most people had nice things to say about the programme and the vets.

On one morning towards the end of that week, Tosca seemed unwell again. I stroked her gently as I examined her and took her temperature. It was much too high – she was clearly very ill. I took her to my local vet to get some antibiotics and an intravenous drip and brought her back home. I set up a drip, hanging it over our living-room door and putting her bed on the floor below it. Mum decided to sleep on the sofa next to her so that she wouldn't be alone.

In the middle of the night Tosca began howling with pain. Tosca was the toughest dog I'd ever known. If she was howling, she must feel awful. I came downstairs to where Mum was sitting with her and stroked her head and her silky ears. She'd had enough and though my heart ached, I knew it was time to let her go.

My parents agreed to take her straight to the vet. Ridiculous, since part of my job was putting animals to sleep, but I couldn't face seeing Tosca go. She had been my world for half my life.

Tosca was always needle-phobic and the last thing we wanted was for her to feel frightened, so I reminded Mum to ask the vet to sedate her first with an injection in the lumbar region.

In the event, that was enough. Before she was given the final injection, which is an overdose of anaesthetic, Tosca slipped peacefully away.

We buried her in the garden the next morning, close to my first spaniel, Bluff, who had died when I was 10. When Bluff went Dad had been redoing the garden with a mini-digger, which made the digging easy. This time we dug the hole by hand, all of us taking turns.

Tosca had been obsessed with tennis balls. They were banned in the house, due to the havoc she'd wreak with them, so we'd chuck the balls back outside when she brought them in and she would grab them and bury them in holes all over the garden. She was great at digging the holes, but being blind she neglected to fill them in and we were forever tripping into her mini-trenches. When we buried her, we tucked several of her beloved tennis balls in with her.

Dogs live short lives, and if you have a dog you know that most likely at some point you will be faced with making the decision to let it go. Even knowing that, saying goodbye is never easy. We were all quiet for the next few days, missing Tosca's ebullient presence and painfully aware of the great big gap she had left in our lives.

CHAPTER FOUR

South Africa

'Is that you, Englishman? I've got a job for you.'

It was my old friend Thys on the phone, an Afrikaner vet I first met when he took me on for work experience as a student three and a half years earlier. I loved working with Thys, but this time I was in South Africa for a friend's wedding, not to work with animals.

I hesitated. 'What's the job, Thys?'

'I've got to implant embryos into six wildebeest. You game?'

How could I say no? It sounded like a fantastic opportunity to try something new. Working with Thys was always an adventure; he expected me to handle some extraordinary situations, to think on my feet and to be resourceful.

'I'm game. Tell me when and where.'

Thys told me to meet him at a junction a few miles up

the road at seven the next morning. 'You can follow me to the farm where the job is,' he said.

I had arrived in Port Elizabeth, in the Eastern Cape of South Africa, two days earlier. As always, the 16-hour journey from London, including changing flights at Johannesburg, had left me tired, stiff and sore, but, as always, the minute I stepped off the plane into the sweet-scented air of Africa, filled with the magical sounds of cicadas, my tiredness fell away.

Minutes later I was through the terminal and into Jacques's arms. We headed out to his truck, where he had a beautiful bunch of purple flowers waiting for me. This was part of the ritual of our many reunions over the five years we had been together.

Jacques and I had first met when I took a gap-year trip to South Africa to work on a game reserve where Jacques helped to manage the volunteers. I had fallen in love with South Africa – the warmth, the stunning scenery, the wide open spaces, the generous, welcoming people and the unique mix of animals that roamed in the bush. And a couple of visits later, I had fallen in love with Jacques, too.

At six-foot-six, broad and muscular, at first he appeared intimidating, but I soon discovered that he was actually a big softie, as well as being hugely knowledgeable, great to talk to and a lot of fun.

For the next five years, all the way through my studies at vet school, we saw one another three or four times a year; Jacques coming to England or me going out to South Africa. I saved every penny I could for my fares, living on meagre student rations, and I organised some of my university work placements in South Africa so that I could combine my studies with seeing Jacques. We knew early on that we wanted to be together permanently, but living and working on opposite sides of the world we also knew that there would be a lot to negotiate and sort out before we could find a way to do that. I couldn't imagine tearing Jacques from the land that he loved so passionately, but neither could I envisage leaving my family and my work to live thousands of miles away from home. We knew that when it eventually came to decision time, though, we'd find a solution. What mattered most was being with one another.

Jacques is an environmentalist. Passionate about wildlife, with a Masters in Environmental Management, he is a walking encyclopaedia of information about South African habitats and animals as well as being an expert in environmental impact assessments – which is now a requirement before any building work can begin on any land almost anywhere in the world.

For the past couple of years he had been lecturing in wildlife management at a local university and he was living in a small two-bedroom house in Alicedale, a tiny village about 70 miles inland from Port Elizabeth and 50 or so miles from the main university campus in Port Alfred. Alicedale was so small it had just a handful of houses, a pub, a convenience store and a hotel backing onto a golf course. The university had a small satellite campus next to the pub, where Jacques taught his wildlife students and which he referred to as the 'Middle of Nowhere' campus.

The morning after the call from Thys I was up at dawn. I borrowed Jacques's pick-up truck, known as a bakkie, and headed for the rendez-vous point. I assumed Thys would stop, but he just hurtled past me and waved. I set off in pursuit, but keeping up was impossible. Thys drove, as he always does, at 100 miles an hour, even on the little dirt roads, some of which wound up hillsides with a sheer drop on one side. I couldn't attempt to match his speed, so I trailed along in his wake, occasionally catching a glimpse of his truck. Eventually I arrived to find Thys waiting for me at the gates to the farm. As I drew to a stop he leaped out of his truck and came over to give me a big hug.

'Well done, Englishman,' he said, beaming with pride. 'You made it; you're a proper vet now.'

Thys is a one-off – a charming, eccentric, talented vet who has been a friend and mentor to me. His skin is deeply tanned to a leathery hide, he has a white beard and an accent so strong that I can't always understand what he is saying. He has spent his life in turquoise overalls, white wellington boots and a safari hat. In his work he sees the occasional dog and does some wildlife work, but the bulk of what he does is looking after cattle on the region's many remote farms. Most of them are more basic than British farms, and some are vast, with upward of 1,000 animals, compared with between 150 and 300 on the average British dairy farm.

As a student searching for placements abroad as well as at home, I had written to several vets in South Africa. Thys had been the only one to answer, warmly inviting me to come and work with him any time. A talented and unconventional vet, Thys may have been past what most people think of as retirement age when I first met him, but he was still a daredevil at heart, as well as a passionate philosopher.

When I first came out to South Africa we would rattle up the red dirt roads in his old truck while Thys talked philosophy and I tried to ask him about his practice. He'd give me a brief answer and then go back to discussing the existential theories and origins of the universe that fascinated him.

When we got to work on the farms Thys got me involved in everything he did and was ruthless about throwing me in at the deep end and insisting that I have a go. It really did force me to learn fast. He took to calling me 'Englishman' and it stuck. All his clients knew me as Englishman, too.

Thys lives on a large farm, also in the middle of nowhere, and in between jobs he used to take me back to see his wife, Johma, who always gave me a warm welcome and plenty of cold drinks and food. The farm is run by their son Johannes, who looks after their cattle and the horses they bred.

Thys also has an exotic collection of pets that he loves showing off. They include a pack of pit-bull terriers, which he lets out at night to guard the farm and which, despite their fearsome reputation, are actually bouncy, friendly dogs; a caracal – a wild cat about the size of a medium dog that has amazing long ears; and four full-grown, extremely large crocodiles, which, thankfully, are kept in a fenced-off enclosure.

An old-fashioned Afrikaner man, from a culture in which men and women traditionally don't have the same status, Thys nonetheless always took real pleasure in my achievements, treating me like a daughter and showing me off to his clients. When I passed my final exams he was genuinely proud and pleased and I was so glad that, rather than resisting change, he embraced it.

That morning I followed him up the long track to the farmhouse, where he explained to me that we were helping out a friend of his with an experimental cloning project. His friend was at the forefront of genetic research and had a raft of PhDs to his name. The embryos had been cloned using cells from the ear of an impressive wildebeest bull and then planted into sheep's eggs, from which the genetic material had been removed. Now we were going to implant them into six young female wildebeest, all at the peak of their reproductive cycles, to see if they would take.

It was winter in South Africa, which meant the days were sunny but mild, which made it much easier working outside than in the relentless heat of summer. Thys set up a table for us to work on and each female, once she had been darted, was gently placed upside down on the table by the farm workers. Thys would then make a small incision down the midline of the abdomen, open her up and locate an ovary. Next to the ovary is the uterine tube, and where the tube meets the ovary there are finger-like projections that capture the egg when it is released from the ovary. Thys placed the embryo right in the top where the ovary was, so that it would be sent down the uterine tube to the body of the uterus, by which time the animal's body would, hopefully, respond and allow the egg to implant.

It was an impressive and delicate piece of surgery and I watched, fascinated.

'Come on, Englishman,' Thys said. 'You need to suture the incision closed and you'd better be quick.'

I sprang into action, closing the abdominal opening with a rather blunt needle so that the wildebeest could be removed from the table and the next one, that Thys was busy darting, could be lifted on.

As we worked our way through the six of them, hot and sweaty from the intense pressure of the work, I reasoned that only Thys could get me involved in something this bizarre.

Finally all six implants were completed, the wildebeest were back on their feet and our work was done.

'Let's hope they take,' Thys said, pushing his hat to the back of his head and wiping his brow.

'Let me know,' I told him. 'I'd really like to hear how it goes.'

'All right, Englishman. Time for a cold beer now. I think we've earned it.'

We headed back to the farmhouse where the owner was waiting with cold drinks, which we downed gratefully before climbing into our trucks and heading back home. The last I saw of Thys was a hand waving from his window as his truck roared away in a cloud of red dust.

Before we headed to Johannesburg for the wedding of Jacques's best friend, I went to visit the local SPCA (Society for the Prevention of Cruelty to Animals), where I was hoping to volunteer when I returned for a longer visit in December and January.

Alicedale is about 30 miles from Grahamstown, which is the nearest decent-sized town, and I'd often noticed the small single-storey building on the main road into the town with the letters SPCA painted in blue on the white surrounding wall as I drove to buy groceries. When I emailed the SPCA head office it turned out that the Grahamstown centre was one of the few with no vet, so they were very happy to have me there. They had Maloli, a qualified animal health worker, and they hoped that I might be able to give him some extra training.

The SPCA serves the townships – areas where poor housing and poverty are the norm. Most of the residents keep dogs, for protection, and most can't afford the prices of the vet in Grahamstown, where the charges are similar to those in England and many times the local wages. So the SPCA, which charges a minimal fee, does vital work.

The day after my wildebeest adventure with Thys I went in to meet the employees there and to find out more about the kind of work they were doing. As I drove into the compound I could see dozens of dog kennels, most of them full, and a couple of cat cages, which looked more like aviaries.

Inside the small office I met the staff of three: Maloli, Yasmin and Liz. Maloli told me he came from a Xhosa family and he lived in one of the local townships with his girlfriend and their son. Short, with a round face and a big smile, Maloli was probably in his mid-thirties. He explained that he spent every day travelling round the townships helping people with their animals – most of them dogs.

Yasmin was a very tall, blonde Afrikaner in her forties. She explained that she went out collecting stray dogs, investigating welfare cases and helping to set up temporary clinics. Liz, also an Afrikaner, remained in the office, dealing with people coming in off the street and with phone calls. All three of them were friendly and welcoming and they showed me around the offices, the examining room, the kennels and the field at the back where the rescued donkeys were kept.

It was good to meet them and I could see that they had their hands full. I was excited – and nervous, too – about joining them in December and keen to do what I could to help.

A couple of days later Jacques and I headed to Johannesburg for the wedding. Jacques and his best friend Eugene, known as Snap, had been friends since they played on the same chess team as teenagers at school. Both of them were talented players – at one point Jacques was extremely high-ranked in South Africa, able to plan 30 to 40 moves ahead during a game. He still plays and he can still see 10 to 15 moves ahead. I do play with him, but as I can just about manage to plan two moves ahead there are no prizes for guessing who wins. It's more a case of guessing how long I can stay in the game.

As a team Jacques and Snap would surprise their opponents. While the geeky kids plotted and planned, Jacques and Snap would go out and party and then get up the next day and wipe the floor with the opposition, who almost always underestimated them.

Snap's wedding to his fiancée Yolandi was in a pretty, rustic, wood-beamed chapel at the bottom of a steep hill on an estate just outside the city. Further up the hill was a lodge that had a lovely garden with a fountain at its centre, which was where the reception was held. We all stood around the fountain as the photos were taken, enjoying strawberry daiquiris and canapés. It was beautiful, but cold! August is one of the chilliest months in South Africa, so I was glad when we headed into the lodge for the meal.

It's the custom with Afrikaner weddings for the groom to be heckled by his friends during his speech, so poor Snap had to put up with the jeers and catcalls of his mates, but Jacques, as best man, had an easier time.

After the speeches everyone danced the traditional Afrikaner *sokkie* dance – a mixture of jive, boogie, swing and foxtrot, which is energetic and lively and a lot of fun. Jacques is a good dancer, but he has size 13 feet so he sometimes finds it hard to avoid my toes and we end up teasing one another about whose fault it is.

Being in Johannesburg was a lovely opportunity to spend a couple of days with Jacques's parents, Elna and Johan, who live in one of the suburbs. I've known them since I first came to South Africa; they treat me like one of the family and I'm really fond of them. Elna is an interior designer, while Johan works for an engineering company. Jacques's younger sister Sonia came round to say hello, too. She works in the law, and like Elna she's warm, chatty and outgoing. Sonia always looks glamorous. As a vet that's pretty hard to do – we spend our lives in practical clothes, with hair scraped back, short nails and no make-up, so I love it when Sonia brings out my girly side and we talk fashion and hair.

It was a short visit for me this time, all too soon I was kissing Jacques goodbye and I couldn't hold back my tears. It would be almost three months before I saw him again, but at least we would be able to look forward to Christmas together.

Mum had warned me that when I got home I would meet the newest member of the family. She and Dad couldn't cope for more than a few days without a springer spaniel in the house, so they'd gone to a rescue charity and found a six-year-old liver-and-white springer called Roxy. She'd belonged to a family that loved her, but they'd had to give her up when they had a baby – maybe on account of her particularly ear-splitting bark, which my parents only discovered after adopting her!

Still missing Tosca, I wasn't sure I felt ready for another dog, but when I met Roxy my heart melted. She was very different to Tosca, in looks and in disposition. Unlike the independent Tosca, Roxy stuck like glue, a little shadow following us around, seemingly constantly anxious. One evening we watched *One Born Every Minute* – the television programme about childbirth – and as soon as a baby started crying, Roxy would get up and start pacing the room. She fussed around Paddy, our Yorkie, too. Paddy was prone to reverse-sneezing attacks, a spasm of the soft palate a bit like a very sudden bout of hiccups. It's fairly common in small breeds with long, soft palates and not dangerous, but every time he started sneezing Roxy would go over and sniff around him like an over-attentive mother.

Unlike Tosca, Roxy was obedient and attentive, desperately trying to please. That is until she went for a walk, and then her spaniel switch flicked on and seemed to short-circuit her ability to hear. On walks she lost her fretful demeanour and became a typical springer, leaping and throwing herself about without a care in the world.

When I started taking her to agility classes she excelled, and we had a lot of fun. She'd fly over the jumps and scuttle through the tunnels. She'd even race over the dog-walk and A-frame. But the seesaw was her nemesis; as soon as it started to tip she panicked, suddenly not quite so brave.

There was big excitement in the Hardy household for another reason, too, because the week I got home both Mum and Ross were graduating. First Ross graduated from Canterbury Christ Church University. His degree was in music, and the ceremony was held in Canterbury Cathedral. Ross is two years younger than me, but his degree was two years shorter, which is why we ended up graduating in the same year. As his big sister I was grateful that at least my ceremony had come first. His was lovely, although unfortunately Mum, Dad and I were stuck behind a pillar inconveniently placed there by the Normans when they rebuilt the cathedral some 1,000 years ago, so we spent a lot of time craning to try to spot him.

Mum's graduation ceremony came five days later in London at the Barbican. Her parents, Grandma and Grandpa Nevison, were there with us, beaming with pride. Mum had gone to art college after leaving school and was working full-time as a graphic designer when she began her studies with the Open University in 1998. After three years she deferred the remainder of her degree to research and write a book, only taking up her studies again in 2011 once she'd wound down her design business. Now she had qualified in humanities with creative writing and we were all hugely proud of her.

Feeling a little left out, Dad joked that his degree was in fatherhood, from the School of Hard Knocks. He hadn't liked school and hadn't done well and when he left he'd gone to work in construction. A few years later he got a job in the City, starting at the very bottom of a large financial institution. Now he's one of a handful of people running the company, though I still don't know exactly what he does!

Before my next locum job I had a couple of days in which to begin planning my trip to Uganda with World in Need. I had met David Shamiri, the director of WIN, through our local church. He came to England from Yemen, and he and his Polish wife Magda do a huge amount of work to help others. In my last year at vet school I decided I'd like to travel and do some voluntary work before settling into a permanent job, so I went to David and asked whether he could use the services of a vet.

World in Need works to transform the world through aid and education, and David suggested I might go to

Uganda to help remote communities without access to a vet to care for their animals – especially goats. WIN had arranged to give goats to many of the villagers, but its aim was to give one to every household as part of the drive to help them become self-sufficient. However, many of the goats' new owners had little idea how to look after them.

So I agreed to go to Uganda for four weeks to help out and we arranged the trip for the following February, after my stint with the Grahamstown SPCA. David told me I would be able to stay with the local pastor, George Amoli. Conditions would be very basic, he warned me, with sparse electricity and a bucket for a shower. And, of course, no internet or phone connections.

'You up to living like that for a month?' David joked.

I hoped I would be. It was certainly going to be a challenge.

David suggested I contact a few animal charities to see if they would sponsor me, and perhaps even donate equipment or medicines. I wrote to dozens of them and eventually ended up in a room with members of the British Goat Society, who were keen to know more about how I'd use their money if they were to sponsor me.

It's probably fair to say that the members of the British Goat Society are fairly passionate about goats. They write the standards for goat shows, of which there are many, and their members can spend many happy hours talking about, viewing and tending to these animals. In the interview room with me were 15 people who were spending the day having a conference about goats.

'Are you any good with goats?' asked one member, peering over her glasses at me.

'Well, I did some work experience as a teenager at a goat rescue sanctuary called Billie's. I learned to muck out and feed and was taught how to trim their feet.'

Home to dozens of goats, Billie's was beautifully run and maintained, and what had surprised me when I worked there was discovering that goats aren't timid like sheep, they're more like dogs and can be very playful – they have big personalities.

More questions followed and I did my best to sound hugely enthusiastic about all things to do with goats. I must have passed muster because, much to my delight, the BGS very generously agreed to sponsor me to put together 100 goat 'goody bags' to take with me to Uganda. They were very excited about supporting a project that they could see would make a real difference to the health and welfare of goats, and hence the owners, too.

I was on my way.

CHAPTER FIVE

First-time Surgery

When I had a phone call asking whether I'd like to do a locum job in southern Cornwall for a week, I jumped at the chance. I love Cornwall and I thought it would be fun to drive down there and have a week in a practice somewhere completely different.

It was only after I said yes that I realised it was, by pure chance, the vet practice where my cousin Kate worked as a senior vet. Kate – actually my dad's second cousin but slightly nearer to my age than Dad's – had married a Cornish guy and they had settled there.

'Come on down,' she told me when I rang. 'It's a lovely practice, I'm sure you'll enjoy a week here.'

So one Sunday evening in early October I packed my bags and set off on the six-hour drive. The practice had booked me into a little coastal hotel nearby, but this time I didn't feel quite as lost as I had during my first week as a locum two months earlier. I was getting the hang of it and enjoying the variety that the job offered, although my staple hotel diet still seemed to be Pot Noodles. My car didn't like being by the sea, though, as with every gust of ocean wind the alarm would go off, so I spent much of my evenings looking up how to turn off a car alarm on the painstakingly slow hotel internet, while repeatedly leaning out of my bedroom window to turn off the alarm, which just kept activating.

On my first day I was down in the diary to operate in the morning and consult in the afternoon. I was looking forward to the challenge of operating, and hoping for something reasonably straightforward.

I arrived bright and early to find that I wasn't the only newly graduated locum who'd been hired.

'Jo! Fancy seeing you here!'

'Oh my goodness, Lizzie, I didn't know you'd been hired too!'

It was a nice coincidence. Lizzie had been in my year at the Royal Veterinary College and during our final year she'd been in the sister rotation group to mine, which meant we had a number of placements together in hospitals, practices and farms as we ploughed our way through the long, long list of rotations on our journey towards finals. And now here we were, the other side of it all, working together.

Lizzie was bold and outgoing, the sort of person who fitted straight into the team and who, after hellos and introductions, was confident enough to say, 'Who wants a cuppa?' and find her way to the kitchen to make tea for the whole team before we started work.

The practice, like many across the UK, consisted of a large number of part-time staff, both vets and nurses. There were four vets and six nurses, plus two receptionists, but rarely were there more than three vets, three nurses and one receptionist in at once.

Lizzie and I had been hired to replace one of the practice partners who had hurt his back – the theory seemed to be that two graduate locums made up for one senior vet. In fact, we soon realised that the practice was overstaffed, and since the surgical suite was about to be refurbished, Lizzie got to work cleaning up and moving items into storage, joking that she was happy to be paid a locum salary to do housework.

Meanwhile I cracked on with the operation list for the morning. Since we didn't have a super-clean operating suite, we could only do what were known as 'minor ops' – those that were less risky and didn't involve going deep into the body – in the prep room out the back.

First on my list that morning was an entropion correction on a cat. Entropion is when the eyelid rolls inwards so that the lashes rub continuously on the cornea of the eye. Very uncomfortable for the poor cat, who gets inflamed and sore eyes. Entropion surgery isn't all that common and I had never seen one performed, although I knew the theory. It involves making a crescent-shaped incision like a new moon beneath the eye, removing the skin in the crescent and stitching the remaining skin together, thus pulling the eyelid back into the correct position. But there were details I wasn't sure about. What thickness of skin should I remove, for instance?

Lizzie stuck her head round the door. 'All OK?'

'Lizzie, have you ever done entropion surgery?'

'Um, no, actually. But Fossum is on the shelf behind reception if you need it.'

'Fossum' is every vet's best friend. It's an instruction manual called *Small Animal Surgery* by Theresa Welch Fossum and it gives step-by-step instructions on how to do every operation you can think of on a cat or a dog.

Every surgery has a Fossum. I took it down off the shelf and pored over it, checking the details of the operation. It looked straightforward enough.

'Nothing to do but have a go,' I muttered to myself, as, with the cat anaesthetised and Fossum open in front of me, I followed the steps, peering across the recumbent cat every now and then to check that I was on course, with a helpful nurse watching the anaesthetic and occasionally turning a page for me.

By the time I'd finished I was cautiously pleased – the cat's eyelids were now in the right place and I'd done a pretty neat job. I asked Kate to have a look, just to check a senior member of staff was happy with my work; she peered over my shoulder, said I'd done well and gave the nurse a thumbs-up to wake the cat. Once I'd made sure that the cat was fine, I closed Fossum, put it back on the shelf with a pat to say thanks, and went to get myself a cup of tea.

My second op was removing two rotten teeth from a greyhound. I was actually more nervous about this than I had been about the entropion correction, despite having done dental surgery before. There had been a difficult practical at university, which became known as the 'dead dog head practical' and which still made me shudder every time I remembered it. During our training we had practised, under supervision, removing teeth from the heads of dead dogs. The first time I did this I had really struggled. The beagle head I had been given – one of many donated to the university from pounds, labs, racing kennels and owners kind enough to leave their dogs for us to learn on – had been used for several practicals before mine, so all the easy incisor teeth had been taken out already. I was left with the outer incisors, which are much bigger than the front ones.

The technique involves pressing all around the edge of the tooth with an instrument called an elevator, which has a sharp curved end and a handle that fits perfectly in the palm of your hand. The pressing weakens the periodontal ligament which holds the root of the tooth in the socket. When the tooth is wobbly, you can wiggle it with forceps to weaken it further and carry on rotating between the two until the tooth is wobbly enough to pull it out.

After 10 minutes of applying pressure, then wiggling, the tooth was still very firmly in place, so I decided I would apply a little more pressure with the elevator, but at that moment it slipped and I sliced all the way up the gum. The clinician in charge came over to take a look.

'Just as well this dog is dead, or you'd be doing some stitching right now. At least you didn't take out its eye. Believe me, that's happened. Now try again, with more patience this time,' he said.

Remembering this, I took a deep breath as I looked down at the very much alive dog that was anaesthetised on the table in front of me. I had scaled its teeth to remove the tartar and now I needed to remove two rotten wobbly teeth before polishing all its teeth to finish. 'Patience,' I reminded myself as I leaned in to begin pressing with the elevator around one of the rotten teeth. I was wearing a mask to avoid inhaling bacteria from the dog's mouth and it was hot and uncomfortable, but half an hour later the teeth were out and the greyhound had a squeaky clean polished mouth.

Two down, one to go.

My final op that morning was an anal gland flush on an elderly pug. Anal gland expression is the least glamorous part of a vet's job and only too common. Anal glands sit at the four and eight o'clock positions in the anus, and if the faeces aren't firm the glands can fill and become impacted. It's the reason why dogs sometimes scoot their bottoms along the floor, and if this occurs regularly the glands can become infected.

The pug was sedated, so I cleared the glands and then flushed them out with saline before putting in some antibiotic drops. It was an extremely smelly job, but just over 20 minutes later I was done. As soon as I was sure that the pug was waking up and was fine, I made a swift exit to get some fresh air.

I began the afternoon consultations still basking in the relief of having done my first entropion surgery, got through the dental op without decapitating the dog and left a pug with a very clean bottom when a young woman in a wax jacket and wellies burst in through the door, tears rolling down her cheeks and a blood-spattered young whippet in her arms.

'It's Sammy,' the woman, Mrs Jones, said. 'She ran into a barbed wire fence, then she got tangled in it and couldn't get out. She's badly hurt.'

Sammy was whimpering pathetically, but whippets and any sight-hound breed such as lurchers and greyhounds have thin skins (and they're also terrible wimps) so I hoped that, once we'd washed away the blood, she wouldn't be as badly hurt as her owner feared.

As I worked to clean her up her owner was wailing almost as loudly as Sammy. Between the two of them they were making it pretty difficult to focus on the problem.

'Mrs James,' I said, in what I hoped was an authoritative yet reassuring voice, 'Sammy is going to be fine. Please don't worry. The wounds are very fresh so we can stitch them this afternoon and they should heal well. I'm going to have to take Sammy from you for the afternoon, and it will require an anaesthetic, but you can come to pick her up this evening once she's woken up.'

Thankfully Mrs James calmed down, and after signing a consent form for the operation, having a last cuddle with Sammy and a final tearful hiccup she left the consulting room. Kate was in that afternoon so she came in to do the anaesthetic for me and we spent the next hour chatting while I carefully stitched Sammy up. Despite my earlier hopes that the injuries would be fairly superficial, some of her cuts were so deep that I had to stitch up the muscle layers underneath the skin first and then stitch the skin over the top.

As well as being cousins, Kate and I had another connection – her parents had moved out to Cape Town, which meant I actually had relatives in South Africa. Before that they had lived all over the world; Kate had been born in Bahrain and they had followed her dad as a family, going wherever his work took them, before finally settling in England for the best part of 20 years. However, her parents had decided that South Africa was where they wanted to retire.

Kate told me that she and her husband Matt had gone to visit her parents and had taken one of the cheap but notoriously dangerous local taxis that pile in about a dozen people along a set route. An argument had developed and one of the passengers had got out a knife and threatened one of the other passengers. The driver had screeched to a halt and yelled to everybody, 'Pile out, pile out!' So they did, in the middle of nowhere, and Kate and Matt had to walk miles to find their way home. I made a mental note never to take one of the local taxis, not that Jacques would ever let me!

I did the neatest job I could on Sammy, but even so, when I'd finished the poor girl resembled a patchwork quilt. She was a young dog, though, and with a little rest and care she would soon heal. Lizzie had taken over some of the afternoon consults that I was meant to do, which gave me some relief and a chance to grab something to eat.

That evening I was exhausted – it had been quite an eventful day – so after a quick supper at Kate and Matt's house, which was so much better than the Pot Noodle I had originally planned to have, I went back to my hotel room and fell gratefully into bed, wondering what might arrive through the door tomorrow. A day or two of routine health checks and vaccinations was beginning to seem quite appealing.

The following morning, as I opened the consulting-room door to usher in the first patient, I was greeted by the shrill screams – there's no other word for it – of a guinea pig. They make great pets because, unlike other small furries, they rarely bite. But, oh boy, do they make a noise when they're excited, nervous, frightened or, I suspect, just for the hell of it. They also hate change, so anything out of their routine will provoke shrieks of protest.

This particular guinea pig, Cuddles, arrived with her small owner, a little girl of about six, and the little girl's mother, who smiled apologetically.

'Sorry about the noise,' she said. 'Cuddles has had on-going problems with mites. She's already had one injection and we've been told we need to repeat them a few times. I don't want Hayley or her friends to get them from Cuddles.'

I looked at Hayley, who had her arm inside the cage and was tickling a slightly patchy Cuddles.

'You're right,' I said. 'Mites can be a real problem. A bad infestation of mites can drive guinea pigs wild – they lose hair, scratch until they bleed and they can forget to eat and drink.'

We'd learned during our training that mites are transmittable to people. There's one mite in particular, called *Cheyletiella*, which gives an obvious sign when you've got them: three bites very close together – we used to joke that it was breakfast, lunch and dinner for the mites. But there are many types of mite out there, and they all present in different ways, with different levels of itching, of baldness and of contagion to people. It's one of the reasons we were told always to keep our arms bare, as mites can lodge in a sleeve or even a band around your wrist. And the last thing you'd want to do is have a hairband around your wrist and then tie it in your hair, covered in mites.

Next in was a large white tomcat, and this poor chap looked as if he was in a lot of pain. His owner, a worried-looking man in his seventies who seemed none-too-well himself, told me that the cat, Charlie, had appeared that morning limping badly and clearly in distress.

'What could have happened?' he asked me. 'Do you think he got into a fight?'

I examined Charlie carefully. As soon as I touched his right leg he yowled and by the way his leg moved around, I could see that his hip was clearly dislocated. It's known as a hip luxation and could only be caused by major force. I needed to do an X-ray to assess the extent of the luxation, and check for internal injuries, too.

'I think he's probably been hit by a car. He has had some sort of impact, and a car is my guess, given that his claws are badly scuffed,' I told his owner, Mr Tindell. 'Either that or he's had a fall. But the car accident is far more likely. We'll X-ray him and see what's going on. Leave him with us and we'll give you a call.'

'Poor Charlie,' murmured Mr Tindell, looking at him fondly. 'He does get in the wars. He's already had most of his nine lives.'

An X-ray confirmed that Charlie's hip was dislocated. The good news was that he didn't appear to have any other serious injuries.

I phoned Mr Tindell. 'We can sort him out,' I said. 'The hip needs putting back but it's not life-threatening and he should be fine. I'll call you as soon as he's ready to be collected.'

I put the phone down and looked at a sedated Charlie, who was being monitored by Olivia, one of the nurses.

'I'm up to my neck in it again, Charlie,' I said. 'I need to put your hip back but I've never done it before. Let's hope someone can help.'

While Olivia continued to monitor Charlie, I went to see if I could find any help. I bumped into Lizzie in the next room. 'Any idea how to deal with a hip luxation?'

'Goodness, no, I've never done one,' she said apologetically. 'You do seem to be pulling in all the tough cases.'

'Mmm. And I thought this would be an easy week. That's what comes of associating Cornwall with holidays.'

'Kate's in a consult at the moment, but when she finishes, I'll take over from her so she can come and help you,' she offered.

'Thanks, Lizzie.'

There was nothing else for it; I'd have to count on Fossum to get me started so that at least I could make an attempt at relocating the hip while I waited for Kate. Thankfully Fossum came through again. There was the description of exactly what to do; you put your hands in this position and then you lift the leg up and push it in, at this angle, with this much weight, so that you can feel it suction into the socket. It looked pretty straightforward. I followed the instructions and got the hip in, only for it to pop out again when we tried to move Charlie back to the X-ray machine to double check that it was definitely in place. At that moment Kate appeared to help. She repeated the relocation steps and when the hip was back she taught me how to do a sling bandage for a back leg so that it would stay in place and stop the cat using the leg while it was healing.

I called Mr Tindell. 'Charlie's hip is back in place, you can collect him in a couple of hours. He's going to feel a bit sore for a while and he won't be able to walk for a couple of weeks, but after that he should be fine.'

Mr Tindell was delighted and two hours later he arrived, cat carrier in hand. 'Bring him back in a few days, just for a check-up, and we'll redo the bandage,' I said as I settled a sleepy Charlie, his rear end swaddled in bandages, into the box.

I wasn't sure whether to feel smug or relieved. I'd pulled off two firsts, with the invaluable help of Fossum and a bit of rounding off from Kate, and so far both animals were not only still alive but doing well.

That evening I drove down to the sea and went for a long walk along the beach. It had been a warm day for October, and watching the sun set over the sea I felt happy. It had its trials and tribulations, but I really was starting to enjoy being a vet.

Grabbing a quick tea break I checked my phone. There had been a couple of missed calls from Betty, whose 12-year-old son Samuel, a very talented and fearless rider, was exercising my horse Tammy for me while I was away. He adored Tammy and I was concerned his mum wouldn't be calling unless there was a problem. I called her back.

'Jo, I'm so sorry, Sam was riding Tammy this morning and she fell. We think she stepped into a hole. She got up again and cantered back to the stables. She seems all right, but we're worried that her leg may be injured. What do you want us to do?'

'Is Sam all right?'

'She fell on his hand. He's got a small fracture but they think it will heal without surgery.'

'Poor Sam, I'm so sorry. And poor old Tammy, too. Don't worry, I'll be back tomorrow and I'll go and see her.'

My last day in Cornwall was non-stop. Eight dogs, five cats, several guinea pigs, hamsters and rabbits later, in came Tito the Patterdale terrier.

A beautiful, wiry little black dog, Tito was gorgeous. But his owner, Mr Hill, looked fed up. 'Tito was chasing a squirrel,' he said. 'He actually caught it, but the squirrel had other ideas about being lunch so it bit his lip. Tito dropped the squirrel, leaped in the air, yelped and came back to me, tail between his legs. There isn't much that stops him in his tracks, but that squirrel managed it.'

'Oh Tito,' I said, stroking his silky head. 'Sounds as though you've been getting into trouble.'

Extremely active and generally fearless, terriers are often terrors. I started cleaning and clipping round Tito's lip, but he wriggled and squirmed so much that it took 20 minutes.

As I worked on him Mr Hill told me he was at his wits end.

'We moved down here from London a few weeks ago,' he said. 'Thought it would be a lovely place to retire, and it is, but Tito keeps escaping out of our garden and worrying the cows on the farm next door. He can get over the wall and I just don't know how to stop him. The farmer's already shouted at him several times.'

'I know what a handful terriers can be,' I said. 'They can be a nightmare to train. But you do need to stop him. The farmer is actually entitled to shoot him if he's worrying livestock. It might be worth putting up a mildly electrified boundary fence around your garden, so that Tito will get a small shock if he touches it. Better that than the farmer shoots him.'

Mr Hill looked alarmed. 'I didn't realise that. You're right, we'll have to do something.'

Tito's wound wasn't too deep and didn't need stitching. I gave him pain relief and antibiotics.

'Come on, Tito,' Mr Hill said, taking his lead. 'And thanks for the warning.'

'No problem.' I closed the door behind them and smiled. Tito was such a typical terrier, lovable but an absolute scamp.

The day – and the week – had come to an end. I packed up, said goodbye to Lizzie, Kate, Olivia and the other staff members and climbed into my little car for the long drive back home. Six hours later I let myself into the house. Mum and Dad were on their way to bed and Ross was out. I managed a cup of soup and a cuddle with Roxy and Paddy and then called it a day.

Early the next morning I headed for the stables to see Tammy. The yard manager said that she certainly hadn't noticed Tammy favouring one leg over the other as she mooched around the field, and as I walked her into her stable she seemed fine, so I hoped she'd got away without any damage. But once in her stable I checked over her legs and I came across a problem. Just above her front right fetlock, the back of her leg felt swollen and warm. I knew that wouldn't be good news, as several tendons run past that point within a sheath filled with synovial fluid. Swelling meant increased fluid, which meant inflammation and therefore damage. I took her across the yard to a flat piece of concrete to trot her up in a straight line. She was about two-tenths lame; only mild damage, but given the structures in the area of swelling, it was a cause for concern. I phoned the local equine practice who knew me and were happy to lend me their ultrasound scanner for the afternoon.

I wasn't an expert at scanning, and I knew I wouldn't pick up on subtle injuries, but even I could tell that a tendon in her leg was torn. She was going to need rest and plenty of pain relief. I put an ice-boot on her leg, above the fetlock, chilling it in the freezer and then wrapping it around the leg and sealing the Velcro fastening. I was going to be away for several months over the winter, so instead of finding someone to ride her, I would let her rest in the field and hope that by spring the injury was healed.

I stood stroking her nose. Poor Tammy, it must hurt. I loved her dearly, but she could be such a frustrating horse. I had first got her 10 years earlier, when I was 15 and she was a pretty four-year-old. Tammy was a bay. Her flanks glowed almost orange in the sun and I loved her from the moment she arrived. My other horse, Elli, had been injured at the time and needed to rest for a year or two before I would be able to ride her again.

Elli had been with me for two years by then and she was so comfortable with me and so safe and dependable that I could ride her without any tack at all, but Tammy was much more highly strung. Nervous around other horses, she would bite the air as a warning if she got scared, and she was so unpredictable that in competitions she would either come first or be disqualified after terrifying the audience by rearing or trashing the jumps.

I always had a bum like glue and I'd been riding since I was five, so I wasn't scared of riding Tammy, and she was bold and learned new tricks really fast, which I loved. But I could never be sure how she would react.

Luckily, despite her wariness towards other horses, Tammy came to trust Elli and by the time I left for veterinary college the two of them were sharing a field at the stables up the road from us and were happy in one another's company.

Despite their size horses are delicate creatures, surprisingly easily injured. With rest and care, Elli had recovered from her injury. Now it was Tammy's turn. I stroked her nose. It might be months before her leg healed fully, but we would just wait, patiently.

CHAPTER SIX

Monday Morning

'Good morning, Mrs Stevens, what seems to be the problem?'

Mrs Stevens, who couldn't have been a day under 80, had come into the consulting room wearing a bright pink mac and carrying a cat cage. She put it down on the table and gave me a wary look.

'It sounds as though you're the one with the problem,' she said.

'Er, yes, I'm sorry, I seem to have lost my voice,' I croaked.

It was horribly embarrassing. My first day in a new veterinary practice, when I was keen to appear totally professional and to make a good impression, and what happens? I turn up croaking like something out of a low-budget horror film. A bad case of laryngitis had left me barely able to make myself understood, to the obvious consternation of practice staff and clients alike. The only ones who didn't seem to mind, thankfully, were the animals.

It all began when I was asked to do a public appearance for the *Young Vets* series, which by this time had been airing for several weeks. My old university, the Royal Veterinary College, asked me, two of the other vets in the show and several of the production team to speak during their open evening. We all agreed and they put us in an auditorium that could hold 300 people. By the time we began it was packed, with people standing at the back and down the steps. The programme had been one of the most popular that ITN Productions had made that year, with great viewing figures.

That evening gave me a little glimpse of fame. We talked about our experiences of making the programme and what we had learned and at the end of our talk we were swamped by teenage girls taking selfies with us and asking for autographs. The first time someone came up to me with an autograph book I was so surprised I had no idea what to write.

It was all good fun, but by the end of the evening I felt hot and feverish and I knew I was coming down with a virus. I was due to begin work at the Dacre House practice the next day – they had hired me as a locum for five weeks,

which was a real bonus as they were a lovely, friendly practice very near to home. I couldn't possibly let them down on
my first morning. That night I dosed myself up with every
cold and flu remedy I could think of, but by the next morning my voice had dwindled to a husky growl.

I turned up for work at 8.30am with my new green scrub
top and my sandwiches in my bag, and smiled brightly at
Bev, the receptionist.

'Hi, Jo, welcome,' she said. 'Glad you're here, we've got
loads of clients booked in and we're really short-staffed
today.'

'Hi, Bev,' I rasped. 'I'll just go and make myself a hot
drink if that's OK.'

Bev looked at me aghast. 'Oh dear. Have you been on
some kind of wild celebration?'

'No, really, I haven't, it just sounds that way. I'll be fine,
honestly.'

I'd been to Dacre House before, as a student. I'd had
several work placements there in my third year and the
practice staff had always kept in touch and told me I was
welcome to come back. So I was delighted when the locum
position came up.

Based in Tunbridge Wells, Dacre House is a family-
owned small-animal practice with a generous and inclusive
attitude towards the local community. They believe

veterinary service should be affordable for everyone, so their prices are low and if someone can't afford to pay they will accept RSPCA vouchers or find them help from a charity. They work closely with animal charities, too, charging low rates to treat rescued animals. As a result they are very popular and are always absolutely packed with clients and their animal patients. And unlike many practices, which use an out-of-hours service for evenings and weekends, the Dacre House vets will see their patients even if it's the middle of the night, believing that it is important to provide a 24/7 service.

The practice was set up about 30 years ago by husband-and-wife team Chris and Sue Murray. Chris, a hugely knowledgeable vet and a skilled surgeon, had just retired, but Sue was still there, though by that time she was concentrating on operating rather than consultations. Sue was chatty, warm and very supportive and encouraging. She told me that when she and Chris first set up the practice they had to sit and wait for patients to arrive. Now it's so full that you can hardly get through the door.

The practice is a converted house, so it's a bit of a maze, but it has two consulting rooms and two operating theatres. Two vets consult every day in three sessions – morning, lunchtime and evening – so the working day lasts from nine until seven, although by the time everyone has been seen and all the paperwork is done the vets are often there until eight or even nine at night.

Several years before Chris's retirement a new partner was appointed. Bradley Curtis was a young, kind and caring vet, a million miles from the middle-aged, rather high-handed and intimidating male partner typical of many practices. Bradley's view was that being a vet is about providing a community service, and he was so nice that all the clients ask to see him.

Alongside Bradley and Sue there was Jane Fairham, another very good and very experienced senior vet, head nurse Emma and nurses Becky and Dee, plus receptionist Bev. There was a vacancy for a fourth vet at the time, which was why I was there. They were looking for a vet who would fit in and were hoping to find someone by the time my five weeks ended.

Back in the consulting room I did my best to assure Mrs Stevens that I was still a fully functioning vet despite my scary voice and, a little reluctantly, she opened the cat box and lifted out an elderly ginger cat.

'Markie's off his food,' she said. 'He's barely eating a thing.'

Judging by his very rotund girth, Markie didn't look as though he was about to starve just yet, but any animal that is refusing to eat is a cause for concern.

I examined him carefully and discovered that one of his nostrils was blocked with discharge. 'Cats go off their food when they can't smell it,' I explained to Mrs Stevens. 'But we need to find out why his nose is blocked.'

Mrs Stevens explained that he'd had bouts of cat flu throughout his life; it had been an ongoing problem for him. Cat flu is usually caused by one or two different viruses and once a cat has had it the flu tends to flare up throughout a cat's life, especially in times of stress.

Mrs Stevens went on to explain that she had recently had painters in the house and Markie had been hiding for days. The clinical signs, plus the history of stress, combined with a slightly elevated temperature meant that flu was almost certainly the problem.

'I'm going to give you some antibiotics for Markie to prevent a secondary infection, which would make it worse, and some anti-inflammatories to help bring down his temperature as well as any swelling in his nose,' I explained to her. 'I'm also going to give you something to help with the nasal discharge. Hopefully we can unclog his nose and he'll feel like eating again. Try warming up his food so it's nice and smelly, or feed him really smelly food like fish, and bring him into the bathroom when you run a bath or have a shower because the steam will really help. Otherwise it's just a matter of rest and recuperation. If he's not improving in the next three or four days, please do bring him back. The next step would be for us to take an X-ray of his nose, just to make sure nothing else is blocking it.'

Mrs Stevens thanked me and left, clutching what seemed like half the pharmacy.

'You OK, Jo?' Bradley stuck his head around the door. 'Heard you weren't very well.'

'I'm all right, I just sound awful,' I said. Actually I felt awful, too.

'Goodness. Well, as long as you can manage. Great. We're full to bursting today.'

I was well aware of that. If I went home Bradley would have to see all the people and animals on the list and he'd be there past midnight. I swallowed another Lemsip and powered on.

Next in was a gorgeous chocolate Labrador called Chip. Bouncy and friendly, he was a typical Lab, but his owner, a woman in her thirties, looked worried. 'Chip keeps trying to chew off his tail,' she said. 'He's really hurting himself. I think it must be itching.'

I had a look. Chip was doing a good job of gnawing at his tail – it looked messy and painful. The skin just above the base of the tail was red and oozy, which looked like what we call a hotspot – in other words, a skin infection. I put a buster collar on him so that he couldn't reach it. These funnel-shaped collars look awkward, but they do the job. Chip didn't look happy about his sudden appendage, but I couldn't let him injure himself. I gave his owner some steroid and antibiotic cream, which works really well for itchy skin, plus some flea treatment because if he had any fleas they would make it worse, and told her to come back in a week if he wasn't better.

By 11.30am I'd seen three more dogs, four cats, a budgie with a sore foot and a gerbil with a sore nose and I felt as though I'd finished a whole day, rather than just the first session. Grateful for a break, I popped home, since it was just down the road, to have some comfort food in a rare patch of late-October sun in the garden. Reflecting on my morning, I was pleased with how it had gone. Despite being busy and feeling awful, I actually got quite a buzz from the intensity of the work, though it was hard to imagine how the Dacre House vets worked at that intense pace all the time.

Back in the consulting room I was confronted with an alarming sight. The guinea pig that had just been put in front of me had an eyeball that was almost out of its socket, making it look oddly lopsided.

Its owner held the guinea pig firmly in place. 'This is Titus. As you can see, something is up with his eye.'

'Yes,' I held Titus's head as I looked carefully at his eye. 'It's prolapsed. He's either had a trauma to the eye, like a knock, or there's a mass behind it pushing it out. Whatever the problem is I'm afraid there's virtually no chance of getting the eye back into the socket again. The only realistic options are to put Titus to sleep or to take the eye out. That's a bit risky because small mammals can be a little bit unpredictable under anaesthetic, but it's the best thing to do. He'll be much more comfortable afterwards and during the operation we'll be able to assess whether there is a mass behind it.'

'Oh.' She looked shocked. 'Well, we'll definitely go for that; we can't put him to sleep. But after the eye comes out will he just have a hole there? He belongs to my little girl, she'll be terribly upset.'

'It honestly won't look too bad afterwards. There won't be a hole; the skin around the eye will be sutured closed and he'll manage fine with the other eye. But we have to get him through the operation first.'

I booked Titus in for surgery with Sue, who was due to be operating the next day, making sure he had a decent dose of pain relief to get him through the night. The operation went well, but afterwards Titus didn't appear to be waking.

The problem with small creatures like mice, rats, rabbits and guinea pigs is that they don't do too well under anaesthetic. The statistics for healthy animals passing away under anaesthetic is roughly one in 2,000 for dogs and one in 1,000 cats, but then it drops to one in 60 for rabbits, one in 50 for guinea pigs and the figures are even worse for small rodents. Sometimes they just don't wake up, and even when they do they are prone to ileus, a condition in which the intestines stop moving, or to getting extremely cold. So when Titus didn't come round as he should have, we were all worried. For a while it seemed to be touch and go, but eventually he woke and after a little while he seemed fine. I breathed a sigh of relief. There's nothing harder than telling an owner that their beloved pet has died on the operating table. I made sure he had plenty of dandelions from the garden to encourage him to eat.

A couple of days later I had another worry with an anaesthetic. We had to do an X-ray on a very friendly Border terrier called Rocky who had a problem with his leg. I had administered his anaesthetic while Emma, the head nurse, was holding him and talking to him to distract him from the needle. Once he was sleepy enough, I intubated him so we could maintain him on anaesthetic gas, but he had taken only tiny breaths, and not a proper big one, in the past 30 seconds.

'Emma, I'm not entirely happy with his breathing,' I said anxiously as she was removing the stethoscope from her ears.

'He's got a wonderful steady heart rate and a good pulse, but I can get Sue for you if you want.'

'Yes please.'

Ten seconds later, Sue popped her head around the door, asking how she could help.

'Well, I induced him and initially he seemed to go to sleep smoothly, but over the last minute he's not been breathing very well. Just a couple of small breaths. Emma's checked the machine and it's all set up fine. His heart is good and his colour is nice and pink.'

'OK, don't worry, I see plenty of dogs that are just more sensitive to the anaesthetic than others and need a fraction of the usual dose. Let's turn off the gas and just leave him on oxygen to flush it out of his system.'

Sue started giving a squeeze of the oxygen bag on the machine every 15 seconds or so to give him big breaths of oxygen since he wasn't taking them properly himself. Two minutes later he started breathing deeply and fully for himself.

'There we are,' Sue said. 'All fine again, now the anaesthetic is starting to wear off and he's lightening up. You can turn it back on now and carry on with the X-ray.'

I was relieved and amazed at how calm Sue was. She had seen this happen many times throughout her career and exuded confidence and experience. I was grateful for her help and I would be more confident next time.

Halfway through the X-ray, Rocky seemed to go the other way; he started taking very large and quick breaths.

'Something's not right here,' Emma said.

I put my ear to his head.

'His tube sounds raspy. Let's change it. It might be blocked.'

Emma turned off the gas and uncoupled him from the machine and together we changed his breathing tube. Just as I suspected, it had partially filled with mucus so he wasn't getting as much oxygen as he needed. Once the new tube was in he settled into a good pattern and 10 minutes later we were done.

The X-rays showed some soft-tissue swelling but thankfully no fractures in the leg he was lame on. I breathed a sigh of relief.

'Not an easy anaesthetic, that one. Clearly just a super-sensitive dog. Thanks for your help.' I smiled at Emma. I wished I felt more confident with anaesthetics. It was one of my weaknesses and I promised myself I would work on it over the coming months.

By midweek I was feeling a lot better and my voice was just about back to normal. No more odd looks from clients puzzled by the new husky-voiced vet! Work was non-stop, but the friendly atmosphere in the practice helped make up for the long hours. Bev the receptionist was warm-hearted, Becky made us laugh, Dee, who was South African, always had a cup of tea ready, and Emma sorted out everything and everyone, impressively keeping on top of stock, staff and animals.

I was grateful for the warm and generous support that all the vets offered. I knew I could check with them if I had any concerns or doubts about a diagnosis or a procedure. That was comforting, because when you're fresh out of vet school everything feels new and there were times when I missed knowing that a friendly clinician was looking over my shoulder.

During your first year as a qualified vet you have to fill in an online Professional Development Record for the veterinary governing body, the Royal College of Veterinary Surgeons (RCVS) – not to be confused with my old university, the Royal Veterinary College (RVC). On it you have to include every single case you see, ticking the boxes for the number of vaccinations, spays, heart conditions, allergies, equine cases, anaesthesias, euthanasias and so on. You also have to write up a handful of case studies and at the end of the year you have to have it all signed off by a senior vet who has seen your work and will vouch for you. Normally this would be done by a senior vet in the practice that you join, but as I was going from one practice to another as a locum, there was no one obvious to do this for me. So when Bradley offered to be my supervising vet it solved a problem for me and I was delighted.

Dinner with my old friend Abi made a welcome break towards the end of the week. Abi and I had been friends since she was 11 and I was 13. We met at the stables and bonded over our shared passion for horses; for years we rode together in the evenings and at weekends. She was the closest I ever came to having a sister – we look alike and we love being taken for sisters.

Abi studied history at university and then went to work for Teach First, the scheme that trains graduates for six weeks and then puts them into tough schools in low-income communities to work as teachers for the next two years. If they make it to the end, they become qualified teachers. It's a great scheme, aimed at ending inequality in education and finding inspirational people to help and encourage kids who might otherwise fail, but the reality for Abi was tough. She is the gentlest person I know, and she found herself teaching seven- and eight-year-olds who constantly needed to be kept in line. She had to look for clever ways to do this, because she wasn't the sort of person to shout.

Although our lives have taken us in different directions, Abi and I always make time to get together for a meal, a drink out or a girly evening in with a tub of ice cream and a film.

She had sent me a text a couple of days earlier: 'Help me, I need rescuing from these kids.'

I rang her and asked if she fancied a takeaway and a comedy. 'Sounds like bliss,' she said.

Two days later, over a curry, I asked her how it was going. 'Let's put it this way,' she said. 'I'll get through it, but I'll be glad when I do. I swear some of the kids have got a diploma in winding teachers up.'

'You're brave,' I told her. 'Animals are easier to keep in line than your little monsters.'

It was great to catch up with one another's lives and, as always, we promised to get together again soon. Not always easy, given the demands we both face, but ours is the kind of friendship that will survive anything. I can see us as little old ladies, still chewing the fat over a curry.

It's funny how animal cases can come in batches. You don't see a condition for a couple of weeks and then three come along at once. When I got back to work the next day the theme seemed to be elderly dogs.

Old dogs generally develop problems. We all do as we grow older, and dogs, just like humans, are subject to a whole range of age-related difficulties. It often requires time, patience and expense to keep an old dog going, but choosing to put them to sleep can be even harder.

Douglas was an old Cairn terrier who had recently been rescued. His owners, Mr and Mrs Miller, had been on holiday in the Highlands of Scotland and the bartender at the hotel where they were staying had Douglas behind the bar. The Millers got chatting to the bartender, who told them that Douglas's owner, an elderly lady, was terminally ill with cancer and in hospital. The bartender had agreed to look after Douglas and the hotel owners had allowed her to bring him to work, but she wouldn't be able to keep him permanently, she explained, because she was soon going to move abroad.

The following day the Millers told the bartender that they would like to adopt Douglas and two days later they drove back down to Kent with the dog settled in the back of the car on a lovely tartan dog bed.

Douglas settled into his new home and was given plenty of treats and love. Everything seemed fine, until he developed a bad dose of kennel cough, or canine infectious tracheobronchitis. Kennel cough can sound awful, as if your dog is choking on something, but in most healthy dogs it's not life-threatening. However, Douglas was elderly, probably around 14, and when his new owners brought him in to the practice he was very ill.

Lethargic and floppy, his chest heaving up and down with every breath, he looked as though he wouldn't last long. I put him straight onto high-dose antibiotics along with medication to bring down his temperature, mucolytic powder to help clear the mucus in his throat and a medicine that relaxes tight airways and opens them up.

I told Mr and Mrs Miller, a gentle and thoughtful couple, to take Douglas home, keep him warm and bring him back in a couple of days. Although they'd only had him for a few months they were devoted to him and terribly upset that he was so ill. They carried him carefully out to their car, promising to nurse him day and night.

A couple of hours later, Sparky the Jack Russell was brought in by his owner, a short, quiet man who clearly loved his dog very much. Sparky, a sprightly little chap of 15, had developed another complaint that is common in older dogs – dry eye. This occurs when the immune system destroys the glands that produce tears and the result is very painful for the poor dog; the eyes produce a nasty discharge and can become ulcerated.

Dry eye isn't curable, but luckily it's manageable. I confirmed the condition using the Schirmer's tear test: you take little pieces of paper, a bit like blotting paper, and insert them between the dog's eyelid and the eye. The paper is marked along its length and it soaks up tears while drawing a blue dye along with it. If the moisture reaches the fifteenth marker, the eye is healthy; less than 10 and there's a problem. Poor Sparky only managed the second marker, in both eyes. I started him straight away on an eye drop that contained a down-regulating drug to stop the immune system from attacking the lacrimal glands, which produce tears, and suggested the owners also use fake tears, which they could get from the chemist.

Sparky's owner wasn't well off and the eye therapy is expensive initially until the disease is brought under control, but luckily, unlike many of the animals that came to Dacre House, the dog was insured. I suggested the owner bring Sparky back in a week to reassess his tear production to make sure we were going in the right direction.

The last old chap I saw that day was an ancient beagle named Bailey. He trailed in behind his owners, looking very flat. Shoulders stooped, ears drooping to the floor, he appeared worn out. His owners, a very charming older couple, said that Bailey just appeared to have lost his spirit. Formerly a bouncy, lovable dog, he had become so lethargic that not even the prospect of food or walks excited him.

Lethargy can be due to a number of conditions, so I did a blood test. When it showed nothing abnormal, coupled with the fact that his clinical exam was entirely normal apart from looking depressed, I was suspicious that he was suffering from a dog version of dementia. Symptoms of canine cognitive dysfunction, or dementia, appear in about 50 per cent of dogs over the age of 11, although in many the symptoms are mild. The good news, as I explained to Bailey's owner, is that there's a very good drug that increases blood flow to the brain, which means the brain is getting a bit more oxygen and nutrients and is stimulated.

I promised to ring in a few days' time to see how Bailey was getting on. I wanted to be sure that his condition had been neurological and not clinical.

Old age isn't easy, whether you're human or canine. All three of my older patients remained on my mind, but one of the nice things about being at Dacre House for several weeks was that I could follow up on patients and see how they were doing.

Douglas came back the following week, his cough much better and his owners delighted that they weren't going to lose him quite yet. Sparky came back, too, his eyes much more comfortable. His patient owner was happy to put drops in his eyes several times a day and just relieved that he wasn't in discomfort.

As for Bailey, when I phoned his owners they said that he was like a new dog, his energy restored and his joy in life undimmed. 'I'm not sure exactly what you gave him,' his owner said. 'But is there any chance that we could have some?'

CHAPTER SEVEN

People and their Pets

'This is Dexter. Our little darling is not well.'

I looked down at the large pet box. Was Dexter a small dog? Or a cat? Clearly he was very precious to the smartly dressed young couple looking anxiously at me from across the table.

Many people become deeply attached to their pets, so I was used to owners being very affectionate towards their animals as well as full of loving concern and anxiety about their animal's condition.

I opened the lid of the box and looked inside. Dexter was a large brown-and-white rabbit.

'Hello, Dexter,' I said. 'Let's put the box on the floor and I'll examine him there. Rabbits can hurt their backs very easily, so I always prefer to get down on the floor with them, rather than risk a fall from the table.'

Once we'd eased Dexter from the box he sat on the consulting-room floor, nose twitching, ears alert. I could see that he had a large swelling on his back.

'It looks as though he has an abscess. They're fairly common in rabbits. It needs draining.'

'But why did he get it? We take such good care of him.' The woman, her blonde bob tucked elegantly behind her ears, looked distressed.

'Well, it could be from a wound – does he share a hutch with another rabbit?'

'Share a hutch?' the woman asked, looking incredulous. 'He doesn't live in a hutch; he lives in our flat with us. Dexter is a house rabbit – he's fully house-trained and very well behaved. And what's more, he doesn't bark and annoy people, like a dog, or disappear at night, like a cat, and he loves a cuddle.' He smiled down at Dexter. 'He's the perfect pet.'

'Oh yes, of course, sorry. I know that rabbits can make lovely pets. It's just that most of the rabbits we see are kept outside in hutches.'

I shouldn't have been surprised. House rabbits are on the rise, an increasingly popular choice of pet.

'As he's in the house with you, and I take it you don't have other pets, I'm not sure how he got the abscess, but don't worry, we can sort it out.'

Actually, draining a rabbit abscess isn't that easy, because the pus inside them is thick, a bit like toothpaste or cottage cheese. And because the abscesses are hard to clear out, there's a higher chance of them returning.

I asked Dexter's owners, who introduced themselves as Callie and Josh, to leave him with us for the day – since he was such a lively rabbit and keeping him still for long enough was going to be impossible, as he'd need to be anaesthetised while the abscess was cleared out and flushed with antiseptic solution. After cuddling Dexter, telling him to be good and promising to be back soon with his favourite carrot treats, they left.

A few hours later Dexter was ready to go home with some antibiotics, none the worse for his ordeal and no doubt looking forward to his treats. Unfortunately he was back again a week later. The abscess wasn't healing and Callie and Josh were not happy.

'It must be hurting him,' Callie said, kissing Dexter's nose, which made him sneeze. 'Is there anything else you can do?'

I decided to have a word with Bradley, so I told Dexter's owners I was going to take him to a senior vet for a second opinion.

'I've seen another one like this fairly recently,' Bradley said, after emerging from the operating theatre. 'I changed the antibiotics and also opened up some antibiotic capsules to put the powder directly onto the abscess, so he's being treated with a combination of antibiotics in a variety of ways. That might do it.'

I explained the change of plan to Callie and Josh, who seemed relieved.

'I should tell you that it's quite expensive treating it this way. The bill could be around £150.'

'That's fine,' Josh said. 'He's worth it to us, we don't mind paying.'

Rabbits can cost as much as dogs or cats to keep; they need to be vaccinated, neutered and regularly given health checks. Arguably they have less personality than dogs and cats, though many rabbit owners might disagree, and they don't live as long. But owners like Josh and Callie, who keep rabbits instead of a dog or cat, don't seem to mind.

Dexter wasn't the only house rabbit I saw at Dacre House. A few days later a giant English lop arrived in the consulting room. A soft, pale grey giant – bigger than many small dogs – and with huge floppy ears, it was a very cuddly rabbit.

Once again I got down on my knees to examine it, wary of injury to its back should it suddenly hop off the table. I approached it carefully – rabbits don't particularly like being handled and are capable of scratching or kicking if they aren't enjoying being touched.

'What seems to be the problem?' I asked the owner, a young woman of about 20.

'Maggie's feet are sore,' she said. 'Her heels look red and painful and she's not moving around much because they must hurt. But I don't know why. I look after her really well and keep all the floors clean. I keep her inside most of the time, but occasionally I let her out in the garden on a sunny day, and I've converted my garden shed into a rabbit paradise for her, too.'

I took a look at Maggie's feet and sure enough the area at the tip of her heels, which should be pink, was red and inflamed.

'She does have sore hocks, but they don't look infected,' I said. 'It's nothing that you've done wrong. Rabbits in the wild hop about on earth and grass, which is soft, so their toes get a grip. Hard flooring pushes the rabbit back on its heels, so they're prone to getting sore. And with a big rabbit like this there's a lot of weight to carry.

'Actually she's a little bit overweight; you need to cut back on her food until she loses a pound or two. Don't feed the mixed muesli type, as most rabbits pick out the yummy bits and leave the healthy bits. A complete pellet is better, with plenty of fibrous hay. I can clip her nails and give her painkillers, which will help. And if you can let her out into the garden as much as possible, and give her a big box full of straw indoors, that will be more comfortable for her.'

Maggie's owner held her tightly while I clipped her over-long nails, but I still ended up with a nasty scratch. Getting injured is an occupational hazard for vets. Cats and dogs can bite, so can small furry animals – I once had a nasty nip from a hamster – while bigger animals like horses and cows can kick and trample.

How can we let animals know that we're trying to help and that if they will only let us, the pain and discomfort they're feeling will almost certainly get better? The short answer is, we can't. All the kindness and care in the world won't prevent an animal from suddenly snapping, kicking or scratching. Which is why most vets, at some time during their careers, have time off due to animal injuries.

My next visitor was a very cute-looking toy poodle called Jiffy who had the worst ears I'd ever seen. She was a fluffy little white thing but you could see the pink inflammation through her ears from the other side. And when I tried to touch them she snapped and snarled at me and tried to bite my face.

Her owner, a glamorous-looking woman in her thirties, was apologetic. I told her I'd need to muzzle Jiffy to look at her ears, but even with a muzzle on she twisted and squirmed as I lifted her ear flaps. I sympathised – I knew they were very painful, but I needed to be able to help her. When I did finally manage to look into her ears, the canal was swollen completely closed, so that I couldn't see down them to make sure her eardrum was intact.

I explained to her owner that I would start with an aural anti-inflammatory to reduce the swelling and that if they came back in a few days' time I'd be able to look into the ear and prescribe drops to treat the infection, as drops would work better than antibiotic tablets. However, if they looked really bad, the only way to get on top of it properly would be to have Jiffy in for an anaesthetic to flush out the infection in the ear.

Ears can be an awful problem for dogs; yeast, mites and bacterial infections can all cause issues and the poor dogs can only let their owners know they're in pain by shaking their heads and pawing at their ears, so a lot of owners don't realise there's a problem until it's quite advanced.

Teeth can also be problematic for dogs. Yorkies are one of the breeds prone to bad teeth; by middle-age they almost all have a few rotten ones, so while I was at Dacre House I decided to bring Paddy in to have a scale and polish. Sue kindly offered to do his teeth, which weren't too awful. I didn't want him to wake up in a cage because he's a terrible worrier and would be frightened, so while he was still under the anaesthetic I put him in a basket next to me. It was after the end of morning consults so I was doing paper-work and phone calls, and once he began to wake I carried him around with me for a couple of hours.

The following weekend was my birthday. It's close to Guy Fawkes Night, so we had a family party with fire-works, all very laid-back and good fun. Twenty-five suddenly felt old. I had the feeling that time was flying by and I still had so much I wanted to do and see. I decided to write a bucket list of things I wanted to do before I turned 30. Once I got going I got a bit carried away and by the time I'd reached number 89 on my list I was beginning to realise that I might just be over-stretching things a bit!

I'd put down everything I'd ever wanted to do, from 'spend a night in a tree house' and 'volunteer in a homeless shelter' to 'explore a shipwreck', 'run a marathon', 'travel first class', 'see the Northern Lights' and 'watch baby turtles hatch'. It was definitely going to be a busy few years!

By mid-November it had been four months since I grad-uated and I was keen to find out what my old housemates were up to. One of them, Andrew, lived not far from me, so we arranged to meet for a drink.

I spent four of my five years at the RVC sharing a house with four boys – Andrew, James, Kevin and John. We had all been in the same student house during our first year and when we found a house to share it seemed like a good idea to move in together. Although we were all very different personalities, we got on well and when, in our third year, we moved from the RVC's Camden centre to their bigger Hertfordshire campus, we were lucky enough to find a house we could all share for the next three years.

James liked the good life. He was our gourmet cook and the weekend would find him creating exotic dishes for his girlfriend Hannah. No student grub for him, he had the foresight to put a casserole in a slow-cooker before leaving for classes in the morning so that he would come back to a real meal, while I, like so many others, got by on pasta and omelettes – things that were quick to make and cheap to buy.

Kevin and John were both from the States, but that was all they had in common. Kevin was from South Carolina and was an outdoor, baseball and hiking kind of guy who loved his steaks, burgers and fries. He missed the wide-open spaces of home and planned to go back after gradua-tion. But John loved Britain and all things British. Clean, neat and organised, he loved traditions like afternoon tea and had shipped his Mini Cooper from the States because he missed it so much.

Andrew was always steady and reliable; an even-tempered, hard-working and talented vet who was stick-thin but could pile away more food than anyone had the right to be able to eat.

Andrew and I met in a pub halfway between his house and mine and spent a great evening catching up on news of our old housemates. James was working in a small-animal practice on the Welsh border, John had decided to stay in the UK and had landed a small-animal job in Scotland, while Kevin was working back in the States and had got engaged to his girlfriend Gabby, a vet who was in the same year as us.

As for Andrew, he'd taken the summer off to recharge after the rigours of our final year and had been doing the odd volunteering job to keep his skills up. Now he was job-hunting, but unlike some of our fellow students, who knew exactly what they wanted to do, Andrew was still unsure. Dacre House was still looking for a vet, so I asked him whether he might be interested.

He said he was, so I put him in touch with them and a few days later he arrived to spend an afternoon with Jane, the senior vet. She thought he was great, and told Sue and Bradley that she thought he'd fit into the Dacre family well and do a good job because he was very clever and a good vet, so they offered him a six-month contract, to begin just before I left.

I was really pleased for him, though Andrew, with his customary understatement, refused to be drawn on whether he was excited. I was sure he and Dacre House would be good for one another and when he arrived, during my last week, he slipped effortlessly into the practice, developing a particular interest in radiology and getting on well with all the staff. He took a share in a house nearby and went back to Dartford on days off to play football and to see his family and his beloved Yorkie, Mac.

In late November, along with thousands of other vets, including Andrew, Sue and Bradley, I went to the two-day London Vet Show – a vast jamboree of goodies, lectures, get-togethers and news about innovations. I caught up with lots of friends from the RVC and went to a lecture on the latest advances in treating itchy horses (Tammy had a condition known as 'sweet itch', an allergy to midges that I was keen to help her with) and another on goats. Many of the experts in the veterinary world are concentrated in one place during the show, so it's a great opportunity to go and hear them speak. And at the end I went home with two big jute bags full of doggie samples, including eye drops, toothpaste and food.

The following weekend I was on call. This involved doing consultations on the Saturday and then being on the end of a phone for the rest of the weekend, plus checking on the inpatients. Some weekends were very quiet, but this was not one of them. The casualties came thick and fast.

The first call was from a young woman who arrived with a small black cat, covered in the remains of what appeared to be white paint.

'My neighbours threw a bucket of paint over her,' she explained, clearly furious and also very worried. 'She kept going into their garden and they didn't want her there. What an awful thing to do. I gave her a bath immediately but being a cat she's been trying to lick off the residue and clean herself and I'm worried because paint is toxic. Plus she stinks, so I know there must still be something on her.'

The smell of the paint was strong, and the little cat, Tilly, must have ingested a fair bit of it; she was still licking at herself. I phoned the Veterinary Poisons Information Service, a very useful 24-hour service, and they told me that as long as the clinical examination showed Tilly was fine, the only thing to do was to clean her up and then monitor her for potential side-effects such as vomiting or seizures.

I gave her owner the choice of leaving Tilly with us overnight or taking her home and watching her closely. She opted to take her home and phoned the following day to say Tilly seemed fine, despite what must have been a frightening and nasty ordeal.

It's always hard to understand people who mistreat animals. Cats wander, there's no way to stop them, and a cat straying into a garden is not likely to do much harm.

Shoo it off, by all means, but to throw paint at it is very cruel.

I was still feeling indignant at poor Tilly's ordeal when a burly chap came through the door coaxing a whimpering young whippet behind him. Casey had pulled off her dew claw so that the quick was exposed. Whippets race around and she had probably got caught on a fence or bush when she was running past. The dew claw grows a bit higher up the leg, so it is never in contact with the ground, but it does have its uses, for instance in helping the dog to grip bones. Dogs can manage fine without one, though, so I gave Casey some painkillers and bandaged her leg. I was grateful that not many people were around, because for the entire 15 minutes that it took to treat her she screamed the place down – anyone listening might have thought I was torturing her. Whippets are not the most stoic of dogs and her owner, who turned out to be a local fire fighter, was amused by her wimpy histrionics. 'Come on, Casey,' he chided her, stroking her head. 'You're showing me up, making such a fuss.'

Once I'd finished dressing the wound Casey stopped shrieking and settled for non-stop whining, which was at least easier on the ear. I asked him to bring her back in a few days' time so that I could check the wound was healing properly, then saw them out and headed home again, hoping to have time to visit my horses. But half an hour later there was another call, from a woman who thought her cat had been injured.

I headed back to the practice and two minutes later she came through the door lugging a cat carrier.

'I'm worried that Pepper might have been in a fight,' she said. 'He was out all last night and today he just hasn't been himself; he's been hiding in the corner behind a chair, he wouldn't come out and he didn't want to eat. I feel bad because I didn't realise he was injured at first, but then I saw that there was blood on his leg.'

I lifted Pepper gently out of his box. He was a lovely grey-and-white cat and he sat patiently as I examined him – until I got to his back leg, at which point he hissed and swiped a paw at me. A closer look revealed several skin-deep wounds.

The thing about cats is, they have a life of their own away from their owners and you simply don't know what's happened to them. Traffic accidents, fights and falls can all cause injuries, so all we can do is try to piece together the story, imagining what might have gone on, but never really knowing for sure.

'These wounds aren't too deep, but they must hurt,' I said. 'I'll clip the fur around them and clean them with some antiseptic. He'll be a bit sore for a couple of days, but they'll soon heal.'

I sent Pepper home with some pain relief and antibiotics. The wounds were almost certainly contaminated, either from when he sustained them or through his licking them since. His owner was relieved and, feeling guilty for not recognising he was injured immediately, promised to make a big fuss of him while he recovered.

The hospital for inpatients at Dacre House is a room with cages along one wall and shelves along the opposite wall packed with newspapers, blankets, litter trays, food bowls and all the other items animals might need.

As the on-call vet you don't have to stay overnight, but you do need to make regular checks on the animals. That weekend there was just one inpatient, a cat called Bobby. Bobby was a timid young Ragdoll cat, blue-eyed and handsome but not keen on attention; he had been hiding at the back of his cage for his entire stay so far. The nurses had created an upturned cardboard box with a hole cut in the front, which he could make into a hiding space to feel more secure. He had been admitted over the weekend for careful monitoring and treatment, clearly unwell, with a temperature that was through the roof, at 40.5 degrees. He hadn't eaten for several days, which meant he was now becoming dehydrated and was losing weight. He had a very swollen lip on the right side, and it was difficult to tell whether there was a bad infection and inflammation there or whether it was an infected tumour. The plan was to stabilise his health over the weekend, starting him on intravenous fluids and antibiotics and feeding him high-calorie supportive food, then, if he was in better health on Monday, he would have a short anaesthetic to take a biopsy of the lip.

I checked on him at about 8.30 that evening, as I was leaving the practice after seeing Pepper, then I popped back at 11.30. Bobby was settled and calm, so I told him I'd be back in the morning and went home to get some sleep, hoping there would be no overnight calls.

Thankfully there weren't, but as always when on call I slept restlessly, worrying that I would miss a phone call. I went back to check on Bobby again at seven the next morning and then headed to the stables to see the horses. I was still concerned about Tammy's leg, and I was applying the ice boot daily to bring down the swelling from her torn tendons.

'Poor girl,' I said, stroking her flank. 'I won't be able to ride you for ages. And without exercise you're going to get even fatter.'

Tammy's weight was a constant challenge; she was always fatter than she should have been and without being ridden regularly she would balloon. She only had to smell grass and she'd put on weight. But the leg needed rest, so she would have a peaceful winter in the field behind the stables and we'd see how it was doing in the spring.

As for Elli, it was time for her annual clipping. It's a pain clipping a horse, but it has to be done because they get sweaty when they are ridden and if their coat is long then when they cool down afterwards, especially in the winter, they can get exceptionally cold.

Elli was generally good about it, but she really didn't like having her chin or head clipped. And unlike most horses, which simply lift their heads up so they're hard to reach, Elli would let me start clipping and then suddenly drop her head to the floor, so that the clippers ended up making a weird line over her nose. In the end I decided it would be better just to clip all the hair off her head rather than try to leave some on.

This time I was feeling arty, so I clipped her initials LE, into her flank. Her official name is Lynwood Evergreen, hence her name. By the time I finished I was the one in a sweat but Elli looked, I told myself with a degree of pride, positively elegant.

I got away with just one more emergency call that day, for a spaniel with a split paw, and I was relieved to have a quiet Sunday.

Before I finished my five weeks at Dacre House Sue got me in to do a morning of operations. 'Good idea to keep your skills up,' she said. I started with a bitch spay and then a mass removal for biopsy before my last patient of the morning – a foxhound that had been eating grass and projectile vomiting for 24 hours. He couldn't even keep water down. He had been admitted as an emergency during the morning consultations while I was busy with my other two operations.

Dogs eat grass to make themselves sick, it's a natural cleansing, but when they repeatedly projectile vomit and do not pass stools, an obstruction such as a foreign body is strongly suspected. An X-ray showed only that his stomach was absolutely full, probably with impacted grass, and there was another area on the X-ray that looked more dense, so we needed to open him up to check for an obstruction.

Thirty minutes later the mystery was solved when a huge ball of grass was pulled out of his stomach and then, from a bit further down the intestines, out came half a broken tennis ball! How on earth it had managed to get that down its throat I could only imagine. And a tennis ball isn't even tasty! But then, no matter how well we think we know and understand our dogs, they can still leave us utterly baffled.

CHAPTER EIGHT

Hoping to Help

As we bumped along the dirt road in Maloli's small truck, heading deeper into the poorest township area, my stomach was twisted into knots of fear. What exactly had I got myself into?

I had flown back out to South Africa the previous week, and after a few days relaxing with Jacques I was arriving for my first day's work with the Grahamstown SPCA. Dressed in a T-shirt, cargo pants and trainers, I was ready to go with animal health worker Maloli on his daily round of house calls.

Once we'd climbed into cab of the pick-up truck I had asked Maloli, 'How safe am I?'

He had looked at me solemnly. 'The townships are not safe at all,' he said. 'But because you are with me, you will be safe.' Nervously I locked the cab door and looked at the sheet of calls Maloli had given me. A long list of brief addresses, consisting of a house number and a township; 89 Joza, 1257 Fingo, with 'sick dog' written next to almost all of them.

The township we were entering was a vast maze of small rough dwellings, mostly constructed from large sheets of corrugated iron, crowded next to one another along unmarked dirt roads.

'How do you find your way around?' I asked Maloli. 'Most of these roads don't seem to have names.'

'If you don't know the townships, you will not find the house,' he said.

Jacques had been concerned about me going to work in the townships and although I insisted he was worrying too much, in truth I was pretty tense myself. All I knew of these densely populated areas was the desperate poverty and that gun crime, knife crime and car-jacking had given South Africa one of the highest crime rates in the world. The figures were coming down, I knew that, but the statistics, alongside Maloli's warning that I must stay with him at all times, weren't exactly reassuring.

There was another side to the story, though. Most of the township people were trying to survive on low incomes and most had animals they relied on, but had no access to a vet. If I could help, I wanted to. Jacques was reassured that I would be with Maloli, a township man himself, and so was I. But I still felt unsure about what to expect.

At my feet was a small bucket filled with the limited assortment of medicines that the SPCA could afford: antibiotics, anti-inflammatories, antiseptic and anti-parasitics, plus needles and syringes and the stethoscope and digital thermometer I had brought with me. That was all I had and I hoped it would be enough.

I'd arrived that morning to a warm greeting from Maloli and the two other staff members, Yasmin and Liz.

'We'll be going in a moment,' Maloli had informed me. 'But first I have to move the cobra that is by the cat cages. If it gets in there it may eat one of the cats.'

I hate snakes, and a spitting cobra is lethal. If it spits in your eye or bites, you've had it. So I watched with a mix of horror and admiration as Maloli put on a pair of goggles, took a long stick and carefully hooked the snake and dropped it into a dustbin. Clamping the lid over the top he took off the goggles and grinned. 'Don't worry. Yasmin will drive it to a safe place, a long way from here, and set it free.' To be honest its freedom was the last of my concerns, but I was impressed that they treated it with the same care they gave all animals.

Our first visit, deep in the heart of the township, was to see a man with a sick cow. We stopped outside a metal shack and I followed Maloli through the gate made of strips of corrugated iron held together with rusty wire. A couple of men, dressed in shorts and T-shirts, pointed us through to the back, where we found two cows inside a small pen with, at one end, a corrugated iron sheet suspended on wooden posts to provide shelter from the sun. One of the cows, a young heifer, had a hind leg so badly injured that she was unable to put any weight on it. She was an Nguni cow, a local breed of small and sturdy cows that I'd come across in farm visits with Thys.

The owner, an older man, appeared and explained that the cows were taken to graze for the day on the common land, or on the roadside, and this cow had come back the evening before with her leg injury. She had probably put her leg down a hole.

The cow seemed resigned, as though she knew there was little hope for her, and a quick check confirmed that her leg had snapped in two. I explained, as Maloli translated into Xhosa, that there was nothing we could do – the cow would have to be slaughtered.

The owner asked if we could make a splint. I told him that even if we could find something to splint it with, a cow is too heavy to manage a splint with a break that severe.

Maloli had told me that there were slaughterhouses in the townships that would slaughter animals and return the meat to the owners, and some owners even did it themselves. I didn't give her painkillers, which in any case would have helped very little, so that at least once she was slaughtered they could eat the meat.

After a bit more discussion back and forth, the owner accepted that he would lose his cow. He took it stoically, his arms crossed. The loss of one cow, when you only have two, is heartbreaking. I wished there was something I could do.

Our next stop was to see a dog that had been bitten during a fight. As I would soon discover, dogs wounded by other dogs were common; we saw dozens of them in the weeks that I worked with Maloli and in many cases the wounds were severe.

This one was a sweet dog, a small brown female with a deep flesh wound in her side. Her owner, an emaciated man in his late sixties or early seventies, seemed fond of her, hovering nearby as I examined her.

In England I would have admitted a bitten animal to hospital and then, under general anaesthetic, I would clip around the wound and clean it up, stitch it and send the dog home with antibiotics. But in the townships that was not an option.

I turned to Maloli. 'Do you have any antiseptic? Iodine? Surely you must have iodine?'

'Yes, I do,' he said. 'Does that work?'

I told him it would help. He produced a bottle of iodine, which I diluted with water from almost black to the colour of tea, drew into a syringe and used to flush the wound. Iodine is wonderful stuff – not only is it antiseptic but it flushes out all the pus, hair and dirt within the wound.

I gave the dog an injection of antibiotics and some pain-relief tablets, but I was concerned that the wound was open to flies and dust. It needed to be covered if the dog was going to have a reasonable chance of recovering. I asked the owner if he could give me one of his T-shirts. I felt bad asking for it when he almost certainly had very few clothes, but he clearly wanted to help. He went inside and got one and I put the dog's front legs through the arms and tied it across her back, covering the wound.

Most of the owners we met were fond of their dogs, despite the fact that in the townships dogs were kept not as pets but as guard dogs, because there was so much violence and crime this was the best way to protect themselves. Many of those I treated were Africani dogs; not mongrels but a hardy breed of survivors that had evolved over thousands of years. The first domestic dogs in Africa were recorded almost 7,000 years ago, and today's township dogs are their descendants. Medium-sized, with long snouts and short brownish coats, they are intelligent and resourceful and are one of the last surviving natural dog races in a world where most dogs have been selected and bred.

Alongside the Africanis there were plenty of crossbreeds, often Africanis crossed with German Shepherds, as many people believed that these dogs were the fiercest-looking. Maloli explained that the more a dog looked like a German Shepherd, the more desirable it was as a guard dog, but pure German Shepherds were very expensive.

Most of the dogs we saw had been given unimaginative names. All the black dogs were Blackie, the ones with spots were Spotty, and there were plenty of Joeys, Patches, Cocos and Busters. They were kept in their compound areas at night, to guard the homes, but during the day they wandered the streets with other dogs, scavenging and fighting over scraps. None of the owners could afford dog food, so these animals survived on leftovers from the kitchen, often a maize-based mush called pap, and occasionally a bit of chicken or burger.

By the time I had been doing the rounds with Maloli for three days I had seen numerous bite wounds, some really severe, where dogs had torn the skin off one another or inflicted deep injuries. All I could do was repeat the iodine flushing and antibiotic treatment and advise the owners to take the dog to the vets to be stitched up, knowing it would almost certainly not happen.

At least with wounds, even deep ones, the dogs had a chance of survival. When I came across broken bones that were very displaced there was no option other than to put the animals to sleep. And there were plenty of broken bones, mostly because the dogs had been hit by cars. On my first morning we saw a dog with a broken back, its back legs completely paralysed. We carried it carefully to the back of the truck and laid it on the floor. A group of children were playing nearby and they ran over, curious about what we were doing. They patted the dog on the head and then ran back to their game. They knew we were going to put the dog to sleep, but the death of animals is common-place in townships and children become used to it. Maloli, who was licensed to perform euthanasia and was very good at it, quickly put the dog out of its misery, then put up the back flap of the truck. It must have been in great pain, but at least it wouldn't have to suffer any longer.

As we drew up outside the next home Maloli turned to me. 'You must watch this dog, he is very vicious.' Clearly there had been trouble with it on a previous visit, but when we got to the gate the dog bounded up to us, tail wagging. Maloli still insisted that we couldn't go inside the gate; we would only look at the dog over the gate.

The owner, a thin man in his fifties, came out and dragged the dog towards us, but it didn't take a close inspection to see that the dog had a great big lump, inflamed and oozing pus, directly on top of its nose. There was no way to tell whether it was a tumour or a burst abscess without getting closer. Given where the lump was I knew that, even if the dog wasn't dangerous, it probably wouldn't let me take a closer look without biting me.

As the owner held it I gave it an injection of antibiotics to get some into the system straight away and then left some Betamox tablets – antibiotic-based tablets that help to control infections – and told the owner to give the dog one every 12 hours, starting the next day. If it was a burst abscess, this would help it to heal. If it was a tumour it was unlikely the dog would survive.

By the end of my first day I felt wrung out. This was the first time I had worked in an area where the people could barely feed themselves, let alone their animals, and I found it tough – not least because there was often little I could do. With no diagnostic equipment and limited treatment options, in many cases I could only put the animal to sleep, or try a treatment that I wasn't sure was going to work.

The following day we went to a very different kind of township area. Townships came in various forms. Some were government housing, consisting of tiny two-room bungalows in neat rows, and some were self-built housing, which consisted of anything from metal shacks to one-room houses, but still with some sort of access to water and electricity. Finally there were squatter camps, which were informal, illegally built, run-down corrugated-iron houses, each surrounded by barbed wire, with no water or electricity. So far we had visited all of these, but now we were in a government housing area, where the houses were built of brick, mostly bungalows, and many of them painted in bright greens, pinks and yellows, although they still had no more than two rooms. The residents here were mixed race, the ethnic group known as 'coloured' in South Africa.

The townships were created during the Apartheid era in South Africa, which lasted for almost 50 years, when black and mixed-race people were kept out of white-only areas. Thousands of people had been forced to live in these crowded areas. Apartheid ended in 1994, after which anyone could, in theory, live anywhere they chose. But poverty had prevented most of the township population from moving anywhere else.

We stopped outside a pretty yellow bungalow and a very large lady, wearing a bright-green dressing gown, came out onto the porch with a teenage girl. The girl had her face covered in a type of clay, commonly used to ward off the sun. It was thick and orangey-brown and looked like a face mask. During my time in the townships I saw quite a few women and girls with these clay masks.

The mum could speak a bit of broken English and, nodding and smiling, she told me how pleased she was that I was there. She was concerned about her dog because it had been doing a really bad job of guarding the house recently; it had just been quiet and had stopped barking at visitors. She took us around the side of the house to where the dog was lying in the shade on its side. It lifted its head up, looked at us and lay down again.

I checked it over and, apart from a little thump of its tail on the floor, it barely moved. A typical lean township dog, its gums were yellow and it was clearly very lethargic. A speeded-up, bounding pulse in the back leg made me highly suspicious that the dog had biliary, known in Europe as babesia, after the parasite that causes it.

Although I had never seen biliary in England, where it's extremely rare and generally only seen in dogs that have been abroad, I had seen it when I was working with Thys. It's one of South Africa's most common infectious diseases in dogs.

Biliary is passed on by ticks. The tick bites the dog and the babesia parasite is introduced into the dog's blood through the tick's saliva. The parasite then destroys the red blood cells, leaving the dog anaemic and lethargic, and because the dog is anaemic it doesn't have enough blood to pump around the system at the normal rate, so it pumps faster, which leads to the pounding pulse in the back leg.

As biliary advances the dog begins to look jaundiced, with yellow eyes and yellow skin, rather than pink, around the anus, gums and conjunctiva. The dog is also likely to feel very sick and, if not treated, it will die. The good news about biliary is that as long as it's caught early enough it's fairly easy to cure with an injection of Berenil, which contains diminazene, a chemical that kills the parasite. I mixed the Berenil with vitamin B to help improve the dog's appetite and advised the owner to tempt the dog with good food and to make sure the dog was drinking, putting a little water into its mouth if necessary.

The owner, still smiling broadly, was clearly very warm-hearted; she cared about her dog and promised to look after it. I told her that it should start to improve within a couple of days, and if it didn't I would come back.

The treatment I gave her dog cost 50 rand, which is about £2.40. This lady was able to pay it, but many were not. Maloli would ask each owner, 'Are you able to pay?' and if they could, they would. But if they couldn't, treatment would still be given.

One day Liz took a phone call from the local fire department, which was located on the outskirts of Grahamstown. They'd seen a dog hiding in the bushes near the fire station for almost a week. Maloli and I dashed over and found a very young German Shepherd of perhaps six months old. Her ears were flat, her tail was between her legs and she was skin and bone. She was stuck in a thorn bush and it took us some time to coax her out with a bowl of food. Maloli caught her using a long stick with a loop contraption on the end, which he hooked around her neck. This apparatus was necessary for dogs we didn't know, which could turn out to be vicious, and we certainly didn't want to get bitten since there was rabies in the area. But this dog, as we soon discovered, was actually timid and desperate for affection.

We got her into the truck and back to the practice, where I checked her over. She was emaciated, covered in ticks and thorns and suffering from early signs of biliary. I injected her with Berenil, dewormed her and picked all the thorns out of her coat. She absolutely loved the attention, timidly wagging her tail and cuddling up to me as I worked on her.

Over the next few days she gradually became more confident, following us around the office. She was nervous about going outside, but we knew that would improve with time. We called her Hondjie (pronounced hon-kie), meaning little dog or puppy in Afrikaans. We all loved her, she was adorable. We advertised her as 'found', but no one came to claim her so she was put up for adoption and went to a loving new home with one of Yasmin's friends.

One morning Maloli and I were called to see another cow. This one was lame in one of her back legs. When I examined her it appeared that she'd had a trauma injury to her upper limb, probably a hip luxation (dislocated hip), which was now back in place. I told the worried owner that the best thing would be to rest the cow, not to let her go out walking or grazing but to keep her in her small pen and bring her food for a few weeks so that the hip would heal and not become displaced again.

'Why don't we give it an injection?' Maloli asked.

'I don't think we have any pain relief in the car, do we?' I replied.

'No, but can we not give it a different injection?' Maloli suggested. 'Owners like to see we've given their animal something, as it gives them hope it might get better.'

'Well, it's just a waste of drugs if we give the wrong kind of injection,' I said.

I had already realised that Maloli's understanding of drugs was limited. He'd had training for becoming an animal health worker, and he jumped at every opportunity to learn from each vet he came into contact with, but in the end he was still very aware that he was not a vet, doing a job that was really better suited to a vet. So what he had been doing to avoid missing anything was mixing together three drugs – penicillin, Berenil and vitamin B – in a catch-all, make-a-sick-dog-better injection, hoping that it would do the trick. Often it worked great, but it was still an excessive waste of drugs.

I did my best to teach him what each drug was for and when to administer it. Maloli loved his job and was keen to learn, he just had only been taught a limited amount of pharmacology as part of his training. Animal health workers are vital in Africa, where there are so many animals and such a shortage of vets, but their training is fairly basic, especially for the job they are expected to do.

Maloli had sacrificed a lot to do his job. He told me that he used to work in another location, but part of his job was to carry out welfare inspections on farms and to give warnings that if mistreated animals weren't cared for, the farm would be shut down. He started to get death threats from one particular farm and it became so intimidating that eventually he had to change his name and be transferred. I was shocked. It must have been very hard for him to uproot, with his girlfriend and their baby, and move hundreds of miles away from his home. But he had, just so that he could carry on with his work.

We were nearing the end of our callouts one morning when we received an extra call. 'My dog has arrived back this morning and its neck is a bit pink,' the owner said.

We thought the dog might have cut himself and needed to be cleaned up and given antibiotics, so we headed over to the house. Before he led us around to the back of the house the owner explained that the dog had been missing for three days and had then returned home that morning, hurt.

When we got to the yard a tiny collie came up and greeted us in a slightly anxious manner, with his head down low and a little wag to his tail as if to say sorry that he had done something wrong. I could see he was nervous, so I crouched down to let him know I was friendly, which he took as a cue that I wanted to play so he bounded the last few metres, his tail wagging.

As he got closer and I saw his neck I suddenly felt I was going to vomit. He didn't just have a cut on his neck – there was a slash so gruesome and deep that he was almost decapitated.

With Maloli translating, I talked to the owner and we came to the conclusion that the dog had probably been trapped in a snare and had struggled to escape for some time, the wire biting deeper and deeper into his neck. It was the most awful cut I had ever seen. I was amazed that he had managed to get home so badly injured.

There was no way that the little dog could survive. Even if the owner could have afforded surgery, it would have been almost impossible with such a deep wound, which was already infected.

The dog's owner accepted the news very calmly. We took the little collie to the back of the truck, said our good-byes and gave him the injection. The last thing to stop moving wasn't the rise and fall of his chest, but the wagging of his small tail.

CHAPTER NINE

On the Side of the Animals

'Do you think anyone is going to come?' I asked Maloli, using my hand to shade my eyes against the fierce morning sun.

'They will come,' he said solemnly. 'Just wait.'

I was still dubious. We had set up a mobile clinic – actually a fold-up gazebo – on a patch of dry grass beside a road in one of the townships so that people could bring their dogs to be vaccinated against rabies, wormed and dipped to get rid of fleas, ticks and anything else that might be lurking.

Along with Maloli and I there were two government assistants who worked as technicians for the state vets. We set up a production line; the technicians were ready to vaccinate against rabies, I was on the deworming, while Maloli was there to help people dip their dogs in the trough of anti-parasitic fluid or to take over from me if a sick dog arrived needing other treatment.

These clinics were held three or four times a year in the townships around Grahamstown. As I was there it had been decided to set up a few extra clinics this time, to try to cover all of the townships in the area. But we were relying on word of mouth to let people know that we were there, so I couldn't help wondering if anyone would actually turn up. Would they hear about it? And if they did, would they bother to bring their dogs?

I peered down the empty street. It had been almost 20 minutes since we had declared ourselves ready and there was no sign of anyone.

Then a small boy appeared, dragging a large sandy dog along by a length of baling wire. Close behind him was a young girl with another dog, this time on the end of a piece of rope. By the time they had reached us there was a steady line of people leading dogs up the street.

We sprang into action. Each dog was vaccinated and then passed to me. I had to open their mouths and squirt in Panacur and then pass them to Maloli, who got them through the dip. Each dog needed to be fully submerged in the tub, otherwise any parasites would survive on untreated areas.

It wasn't easy. Some dogs were compliant, others not keen at all, but we got them through the production line at the brisk rate of one a minute. A large crowd of children stood watching us, fascinated by what we were doing. One little boy, a lovely bright-eyed child with a big smile, decided he would help me. As each dog came along he grabbed it and opened its mouth for me. He spoke only a few words of English, but he told me his name was Mati and we smiled and nodded to one another. He couldn't have been more than eight years old but he did a fantastic job; he wasn't at all afraid of the dogs and I liked to think that he might be a future vet in the making.

As the morning wore on the dogs kept coming; a non-stop stream of them, brought mostly by children who yanked them along using wire, chains or rope. We worked well and although it was tough going, my only real concern was that there were no rubber gloves available, which meant getting the saliva of all those dogs on my hands. Rabies was a real problem in South Africa because so few dogs were vaccinated, hence the clinic, and if any of those dogs we treated already had it, any broken skin on my hands would put me at real risk. I had been vaccinated against rabies before I left England, but like any vaccine it is not 100 per cent effective and the advice is that if you are exposed to rabies you should have another course of vaccinations. I just hoped I wouldn't need it.

Every now and then a dog was brought along that was obviously sick or injured. I would break off from worming, handing over to Maloli, and take the dog to one side to examine it. Most of those that were ill were lethargic and showing signs of biliary, so I treated them with an injection of Berenil and advised whoever brought the dog along, often a child of nine or ten, to let the dog rest in the shade, since many dogs had no shade or had a tin kennel in the sun, and to feed it, make sure it had water and to phone the SPCA if it wasn't improving in a few days so we could recheck and possibly repeat the treatment.

Towards the end of the morning a young boy appeared with a Staffordshire bull terrier, another breed that was fairly popular. This little dog had clearly been burned; he had open wounds on his back and was in a bad state. The boy told me, through Maloli, that a man who had a dispute with his father had poured boiling water over the dog. I was horrified that someone could purposely make an animal suffer so badly. I gave the dog antibiotics, a couple of days' pain relief and sprayed the damaged areas of skin with an antiseptic wound spray. There was little more I could do – I only hoped it would be enough to ease the dog's pain and allow its wounds to heal.

By the time we finished we were hot, tired, filthy and very pleased; we must have treated between 200 and 300 dogs. Maloli and I piled the gazebo and all the equipment into the back of the truck, took it back to the SPCA offices and stored it away carefully, ready for the next clinic the following day. Then we went out on our rounds, catching up with several urgent cases. By midday the sun was baking and the pick-up truck was like an oven. I loved the sun, but I wasn't used to working in that kind of heat day after day, so I was thankful to get back to Jacques's house for a long shower and a very cold drink.

It was early January, midsummer in South Africa, and I was back with the SPCA after a Christmas break. I'd taken a couple of weeks off so that we could spend Christmas with Jacques's parents at their holiday home in Groot Brak, a small village on the coast near the harbour town of Mossel Bay on the Southern Cape, on what's called the Garden Route. It's a beautiful area, with miles of unspoilt beaches. For us it was a 400-mile drive, but for Jacques's parents it was 750 miles from their home in Johannesburg. It's a vast distance to travel for a holiday break – to put it in perspective, Land's End to John O'Groats is only 600 miles – but in South Africa it's the norm to drive for many hours to get to where you need to be.

Jacques and I actually took four days to get there because, being the romantic that he is, he decided to take me via the Baviaanskloof Nature Reserve. It's a vast mega-reserve stretching over more than a thousand square miles of mountainous, rugged wilderness. The drive through the mountain pass is stunning, the endless views completely unspoilt.

We set up camp each day and then spent our time hiking up the mountains and swimming in the rivers and at night we sat outside our tent and looked at the stars, which, without any light pollution, filled the clear night sky. It was idyllic and apart from a few baboons and buffalo, there were not many animals about so we could relax and enjoy walking in the open without worrying.

When we reached Groot Brak, after a long, hot drive, it was lovely to see Elna and Johan and a couple of days later, on Christmas Eve, Jacques's sister Sonia arrived to join us.

Jacques and I had to rush out and do our Christmas shopping at the last minute. I love Christmas and I'm normally prepared way in advance. I like making my own presents – things like lavender candles, eucalyptus and mint foot scrubs and spice mixes for different types of meat – but, much to my dismay, my luggage had been too heavy and I'd had to leave all the presents for Jacques's family behind in England. Jacques always leaves it to the last minute anyway, so Christmas Eve found us racing around the shops of Mossel Bay, trying to find the right gift for each person. Needless to say, both of us were pretty fed up with shopping by the end of the day.

I'm used to cold English Christmases and a big family affair, with lots of relatives arriving, a full turkey lunch, mince pies, games and a fire burning in the grate. But in South Africa, Christmas Day was somewhat different. It started at midnight, when we opened our presents before bed, to avoid distracting from the real meaning of Christmas the following day. Then early in the morning we went as a family for a Christmas church service, but being in Afrikaans, most of it went over my head. At least I could sing the hymns I knew in English while the rest of the congregation sang in Afrikaans. For lunch it was cold *turducken* – turkey, duck and chicken – salad and a walk on the beach afterwards. It was lovely, but no matter how hard I tried to feel the spirit of it, it just didn't feel like Christmas.

I was beginning to feel pretty homesick, so I was looking forward to seeing Mum, Dad and Ross on Skype that afternoon. But it turned out the local phone tower had gone down, so there was little to no internet. I just managed to connect and then the screen froze and all I could hear was Dad saying, 'At least the picture froze with you smiling,' which made me cry because I missed them so much.

The week after Christmas was lovely. We ate lots, wandered around markets, tried mini-golf (I lost) and went on a treetop zip-wire adventure in which Jacques kept telling me to 'hurry up' as I plucked up the courage to jump off each platform and slide along the zip wire to the next one, 30 feet above ground. I'm normally scared of heights, but I was so busy focusing on what I had to do and telling Jacques to back off and let me do it in my own time that I forgot to notice just how high we were.

One evening we went to a beach restaurant which served a 10-course, all-you-can-eat seafood buffet. They told us to bring our own wine and leave our shoes in the car and all the food was cooked over a fire in front of us. It tasted wonderful and we had a great night, although the owners might have wished they'd thought twice about the all-you-can-eat part once Jacques got stuck in. The chefs were clever, though, and served delicious and very filling home-made bread with the first course. I was warned 'beware of the bread', and several courses in I understood why.

On New Year's Eve we watched the crazy illegal firework display on the beach and had a glass of champagne. I was sure that 2015 was going to be a wonderful year for both of us. I knew I'd found the right man in Jacques and I hoped we'd begin working out how to bring our lives together from opposite sides of the world. I knew he felt the same way, but I worried sometimes that he seemed reluctant to talk about the practical aspects of being together. Whenever I raised the topic of which of us would move countries he said we could think about it later. But when would that be?

With Christmas and New Year over we headed home via the Karoo National Park, a starkly beautiful mountainous desert 200 miles north of Mossel Bay. We spent two nights camping there and it was so hot that we had to stay in the car with the air-conditioning on or lie in the little shade that there was, or swim in the pool at the campsite. On our first full day we started preparing some food for a *braai* – a South African barbecue. Jacques asked me to go into the tent to get some ingredients, but when I lifted the flap I got a shock. Jacques had left his cold damp towel in the tent and it had attracted an army of red ants. They had gnawed through the groundsheet and infested the tent so that everything in it was covered by a rustling, shifting blanket of ants. I screamed and ran, so poor Jacques had to take everything out of the tent, shake off the ants, dozens of which bit him, and move the tent, all in 40-degree heat! He wasn't too happy with me.

After that we decided that eating at the campsite restaurant would be a much easier option, which turned out to be just as well because a massive thunderstorm appeared out of nowhere. Half an hour of torrential rain left the most incredible sky, and Jacques's irritation with me for leaving him to fight off the ants alone soon dissolved as he stood behind me, wrapping me in his arms, and we just looked up in awe at the explosion of vibrant colours in the sky.

From Karoo we drove to the Valley of Desolation, a sheer 400-foot cliff face, formed over millions of years, which has been declared a national monument. Karoo is famous for its extraordinary storms and as we drove we could see that a huge thunderstorm was gathering to one side of us. 'Look over there,' Jacques said, turning towards the other side. I gasped; there was a vast sandstorm. For the next few miles it looked like the apocalypse, with dark clouds of sand whirling on one side and huge bolts of lightning shooting down from a black sky on the other. We kept driving, hoping we could pass between them before the two met.

Suddenly we realised the tarpaulin on the back of the truck had come loose and was flapping wildly in the wind. If we didn't secure it, it would blow away or our luggage underneath would get drenched or fly off. Jacques stopped the car in a spot where the road cut through a small hill, to give us some protection, and opened the car door, which was almost ripped off by the wind. He is a big man, built like a rugby player, standing at exactly two metres high, but when he got out he was almost blown off his feet and he struggled for several minutes to secure the tarpaulin. The next challenge was to retrieve his hat, which had been swept off his head. In the end he gave up and, leaning diagonally into the wind, fought his way back to the car.

We made it through the storms and spent a night in a guest house, which was bliss – no ants, no canvas and nice bathrooms. That evening, after the storms had calmed down and before night drew in, we drove to the top of the valley to watch the sunset and as we stood in its red glow Jacques said, 'Wait, I forgot something,' and reached for a small, square object in his pocket. My heart leaped. Had he chosen this wonderful spot to propose? For a split second I waited – until he pulled out his GoPro camera, turned to me and said 'Selfie!' I sighed. It was a bit of a running joke between us that I was waiting for him to propose and I was beginning to wonder if he would ever actually do it.

The week we got back to Alicedale I was due back at the SPCA, but the rain came down in torrents, the dust roads turned to thick mud and it became impossible for me and Maloli to get into the townships.

When the rain finally eased off and the roads were passable again we got back to work, setting up the mobile clinics and continuing with our house visits. One of the first animals I saw was a little grey donkey that had been hit by a car. He had a soft-tissue pelvic injury which I thought might heal – if the owner would allow the donkey to rest for a couple of months. The township people could only afford animals that worked to earn their keep, so the concept of allowing an animal to rest was an alien one and it took a great deal of persuasion to get the owner, who used the donkey to carry cans of fuel that he sold, to rest him. My heart broke for the little donkey. I felt very unsure that the owner really would keep his word.

Many of the cases I saw I was never able to follow up on, but in this case Maloli went back a few weeks later and he told me that the man had rested the donkey and it had recovered, much to the owner's delight, which was lovely news. I got the impression the owner would treat his donkey with more respect now and give him a break every now and then.

Not many cases within the townships were happy ones. The level of poverty was very high, and animals certainly weren't respected or treasured, so many were left suffering. It was also a prime hot spot for the quick spread of diseases, particularly in dogs, since all dogs intermingle during the day and none are vaccinated unless they have been seen at one of the SPCA clinics, and even then, vaccines only last a year. One of the saddest cases I came across was a litter of five very pretty puppies, all of which had parvovirus – a highly contagious and lethal disease. Almost all dogs in England are vaccinated against parvo, so I hadn't seen it before, but I recognised the symptoms: rapid weight loss, lethargy and haemorrhagic diarrhoea. The dogs rapidly become weak and dehydrated and usually died within a few days. The owner said he had already lost two puppies over the previous two days.

In some cases, if a dog is kept in isolation and nursed carefully and intensively with intravenous fluids and round-the-clock care, it can recover. But for these puppies that wasn't possible – the owners couldn't look after them and the SPCA didn't have any isolation facilities, so the only option was to put all the puppies to sleep. A heart-breaking job, which left me feeling very sad.

A day or two later we rescued another litter of puppies, lovely little sandy-coloured creatures. The owner couldn't afford to feed them, so we took them to the SPCA, hoping to find homes for them, but there was an outbreak of parvovirus in the kennels and so we lost them all as well. It was devastating to lose so many puppies in such a short space of time.

On our round of house calls there was often a need for improvisation to use whatever we had to hand to treat the animals. When we went to see a big dog with an abscess on the side of its face I knew I'd get my hand bitten if I tried to take a closer look. Maloli refused to get near the dog, having been bitten by him once before, and I didn't have a muzzle. The abscess needed draining, so I asked the teenage boy who was the only person at home if he had anything soft I could use to tie the dog's mouth shut.

He disappeared and came back with a rugby sock, which he tied around the dog's nose. But as the dog growled, the boy got frightened and let go and I had to whip my hand out of the way of its jaws. I took the sock, wrapped it around the dog's muzzle, crossed it over under his chin and pulled it tight behind his ears, so the boy could hold it there without being scared and stop the dog from moving backwards.

It worked really well and I was able to treat the dog's abscess, showing Maloli how to drain it and hopefully giving the dog some relief. Maloli, the boy and several onlookers who had gathered round were impressed with my bravery, but as I explained to Maloli afterwards, it was less heroic bravery and more a case of having to make a plan because I was quite keen on keeping all my fingers.

Scalded animals became another theme. I was shocked and saddened by how often animals suffered the consequences of disputes between neighbours or rivals. As I treated a dog with serious burns in one front yard, a man came out of the next house and said would I look at his donkey, which had also been scalded with hot water? The wounds weren't new, the injury had clearly happened a few days earlier. The donkey must have been in terrible pain.

'Who did this?' I asked him.

'The man in that house over there,' the owner said, pointing at a shack across the street. 'He does not like me.'

'That's hardly your donkey's fault,' I muttered. Animals were seen simply as possessions and it was deeply upsetting.

I had become a vet to help animals, to end their pain and suffering, to heal their wounds and diseases and to restore them to health. And while there will always be animals too ill or too injured to help, back in England in most cases I can do something to make the animal better. In the South African townships, though, I had to face a much harsher reality. Animals were kept not as pets but to work or guard the house, and since the owners were often too poor to feed themselves properly, they simply couldn't afford treatment for their animals. Anything over the equivalent of £4 was out of the question for most people and the result was that many animals died that could have been saved.

At least with wounded animals disinfecting the wound and administering antibiotics gave many of them a good chance of survival. I saw several that had nasty cuts on their necks from the wire so often used as a collar and most of them could be saved. But some injuries were impossible to treat. Among them was a little terrier that Maloli and I went to visit in one of the roughest township areas. We were shown into a small yard where the dog lay in a patch of shade looking pitiful, her eyes pleading. When I got close and saw her injury I felt my stomach turn over. Her foot was so badly broken that all four toe bones were sticking out through the skin. I knelt and stroked her head. 'You poor thing,' I murmured. 'How long have you been like this? I wonder what happened to you.'

Maloli asked the owner, a young girl of about 15, what had happened, but she didn't know. She suspected that the dog had been hit by a car, which was an all-too-common scenario in the townships. As was so often the case, the dog had been injured while out on her own and had come home in this state – though how she managed to walk I can't imagine.

I explained that there was no possibility of repairing this damage and the dog was in great pain. I would need to put her to sleep, straight away.

Many owners, when we broke this news, were resigned and accepted it calmly. But the girl looked horrified and spoke rapidly to Maloli. I knew she was asking if there was any way to save her dog, who she said was called Halala, which means happy in Xhosa. Maloli translated and when I said that I was very sorry, but the dog could not be helped, tears ran down the girl's cheeks. She sat and stroked Halala, whose tail thumped softly on the ground, before Maloli picked her up and gently carried her to the truck. I followed and when I looked back the girl was still sitting on the ground in the yard, wiping tears from her eyes.

One afternoon Maloli and I went to inspect a pig farm. Part of his job, in addition to house visits, was inspecting premises where animals were bred. The SPCA had received a complaint about this particular farm, so we went to see what was going on.

The scene that greeted us was worse than I could have imagined. The pigs were being kept in several small pens made of rusty metal, each about four feet by six and most knee-deep in mud and muck. Some had corrugated-iron roofs, which provided little protection; others had no roof at all and the pigs, crowded together, were helpless in the hot sun. Worst of all, none of the pens had food troughs in them and only a few contained a water bucket. Overcrowded, hot, dehydrated and hungry, the pigs were in a pathetic state. About 20 men from the local townships had put this together as a kind of farm cooperative. They bred pigs and sold the piglets in the townships for families to raise for their meat.

There was not a lot of money changing hands, most of the piglets were exchanged for goods, which meant they had little money to spend on improving conditions.

Maloli had to tell them that their pigs would be taken away if the men didn't make brick pens with shade, food and water. The men argued with him and gesticulated a lot, but he held his ground and in the end they walked away.

'They say they will do it,' he said as we got back into the truck. 'I have told them we will come back in two weeks.'

I wasn't keen to return to the farm with Maloli, given that he was regularly threatened when he told people they could be prosecuted on welfare grounds and have their animals taken away. But in the end I had to go with him since it would use extra petrol for him to come back to the SPCA to pick me up before going on the daily rounds. This time there were even more men and some of them looked menacing, so I refused to get out of the car. Maloli went and talked to them and there was a lot of shouting, but when he came back he was pleased. They were going to start building some pens, he said. They would get some discounted bricks from the quarry next door and they had agreed to build a certain number of pens each month. Maloli would need to keep going back to check on them, but it was a start.

Incidents like this made me realise just how brave Maloli was. He was just one man, with no weapon or back-up, confronting a group of men who looked aggressive and some of whom visibly brandished sticks, never mind what weapons they might have hidden. He was threatening to take away their business and they didn't like it, but Maloli did it anyway. He refused to be intimidated. He was on the side of the animals and he was not about to let them down.

CHAPTER TEN

The Handprint

One hot afternoon in mid-January I had a half-day at the SPCA, which was nice because it meant I would be back home by mid-afternoon and have a few hours before Jacques finished work.

I decided to clean up the house, which had become a bit chaotic, with both of us working.

As a treat I put some muffins in the oven to have once I'd finished, and to welcome Jacques home.

I liked things neat and tidy and Jacques was the complete opposite, so there was quite a lot to clear up, but an hour later the house looked great and Jacques walked in with a 'Honey, I'm home', gave me a kiss and grabbed a muffin from the rack.

'Ouch!' he said, rushing for the cold tap.

'Um, I was just going to mention that they've only just come out of the oven,' I said.

Once he'd finally finished his muffin, I could see he wanted to ask me something. Whenever he wanted a favour he would turn super sweet, putting on a schoolboy grin and coming to give me a hug.

'Baaaaaaaaaby. You know you love me?'

'Uh-huh. What do you want?' I asked dubiously.

'Well, work is doing this community project where all the staff and students are making tiles out of salt dough and pressing handprints into them so that the kids in the township can paint them and turn them into a wall. I think it's meant to resemble some kind of togetherness. Anyway, I need to make some tiles. Can you help?'

I was always happy to do things like this. I liked community work, and this sounded like a lovely idea. 'OK, sure, what can I do?'

'Well, I can make the dough, but my hands are ridiculously huge and I don't think my handprint will fit on the size of tile I have to make, so can you press your hand in?'

We did our best to make the tiles to the specification Jacques said they needed to be, with him standing behind me and helping me press my hand hard into them to get a decent shape. They actually looked pretty good. We put them in the oven, which was still cooling after the muffins, to harden overnight.

While I made a quick pasta supper Jacques, apologising and promising he'd wash up, nipped out to collect some work he'd left with a friend.

The next day, I was on my way back home from the SPCA when I remembered that we had no food in the flat for supper. Jacques had been working really long hours the past few days, so he hadn't had a chance to shop either. Hot and tired after more than 15 house calls, I couldn't face stopping off at the supermarket.

I rang Jacques. 'Fancy going out for a pizza tonight?'

He loved the idea and as our favourite pizza place was close to our special spot, on the dunes behind the beach, he suggested we go there first to sit and watch the sunset. I had been in South Africa for a month and a half and we hadn't yet found an opportunity to go to the place we both thought of as uniquely ours, so I was delighted.

Once we'd both had showers and changed, we headed off. Jacques had picked up some quiches and brownies from my favourite café for us to snack on and I was looking forward to relaxing on the sand as the temperature sank from fierce heat to the balmy cool of the evening.

When we got to the beach we left our shoes in the car and started trekking up the sand dune. Our special spot was an extraordinary place. We'd come across it on a walk one day when we had just started dating and decided that this was where we would always come to be together and enjoy the beauty of the view. It was an opening between the green bushes right on the top of a very large sand dune, covered with wild lilac coastal flowers.

To the left you could see several miles up the deserted white sand beach with its lush green dunes. To the right you could see for a couple of miles until the dunes became more like cliffs, full of hidden coves. And out in front stretched the sea. It was a prime spot for dolphins and a migration route for southern right whales. If you came when it was getting dark, you'd see the chokka boats far out at sea, shining bright lights into the water to catch squid. Needless to say, the calamari in the area was a speciality.

It was a beautiful evening; there was a slight breeze, the sun was going down and the sky was filled with pink and gold. The beach was deserted in both directions and there was a school of dolphins playing in the water in front of us. We laid out a blanket and snuggled up together, watching the dolphins, chatting and eating the food Jacques had brought.

'I've got a present for you,' Jacques said.

'Really?' I was puzzled. 'It's not my birthday, Christmas is over, what's the occasion?'

Jacques grinned and passed me a square box with

pictures of us together on the lid. It was lovely and I couldn't wait to open it.

I undid the clasp and opened the lid. Inside was a salt dough tile with my left handprint on it.

As I stared at the salt tile, puzzled, I suddenly realised what was different about it. A beautiful Celtic diamond ring was pressed into the salt dough on the fourth finger of my left handprint. It was more beautiful than I had ever imagined, I couldn't take my eyes off it.

There was a moment's silence and then ...

'Yes,' I said. 'Yes, yes, yes.'

'Hey, hang on a moment, I haven't asked you yet,' Jacques joked. 'I was waiting for you to look at me.'

I laughed. 'Sorry.'

He took the ring out of the tile, attempted to get onto one knee in the deep sand and stared into my eyes. 'Will you marry me?'

'Absolutely yes!' He put the ring on my finger and I couldn't stop smiling. It fitted perfectly.

'You know, you could have stood up so I could do the one knee thing properly,' he added.

'Jeez, do you want me to say yes three times?'

He laughed and said no, it was OK but he would have to tell everyone that I did it all wrong. I punched him on the arm. 'Don't you dare!'

I was ecstatic. I was going to marry the love of my life.

I had a thought. 'The salt tiles – were they actually for a community project, or was it all a cunning ploy?'

'Yes, it was,' he said. 'A ploy, that is.'

'I can't wait to tell my parents! They'll be so happy!'

'They know. I didn't go to a colleague's house last night. I went to Skype them to ask permission. I think I was more nervous doing that than this.'

He is such a gentleman. Thousands of miles away, and in an age when asking parents' permission is rare, he still thought it was important. His chivalry is one of the reasons why I love him so much.

Jacques had gone to so much trouble. Got my handprint, chosen the ring I'd always dreamed of and made the box, putting pictures of us on the top.

It was a romantic moment that I will always remember: our special place, the sunset, the ring, and Jacques, teasing me mercilessly.

The following evening we celebrated with a group of good friends in Louis's Pub, next door to Jacques's flat. Louis was a vibrant old Afrikaner, grey-haired, with a big moustache and a thick Afrikaans accent. He ran the pub with his wife Kareen; she worked behind the bar and Louis shared bar duties and cooked. There was no set menu, Louis would just cook something when you asked him to, and it would always be good. Relaxed and easy-going, the two of them knew most of the clients who came in and our friends would often meet there.

That evening we sat on benches outside around the fire, drinking champagne.

'Finally decided to tie the knot, eh?' said Bruce, one of Jacques's closest friends.

'Yup,' said Jacques, smiling at me. 'Can't think why, but I did.'

'Your hilariousness must be the reason I said yes,' I said as I pushed him sideways so he nearly fell off the end of the bench we were sitting on.

'You've got a lifetime with her, Jacques. You better watch out,' Bruce interjected. 'Let's toast the happy couple. May you have a lifetime of happiness, laughter and blessings. Or at least a good few years before you annoy each other to death. To Jacques and Jo.'

'Jacques and Jo!' the group shouted, raising their glasses.

'Now let's all have some shots,' Bruce insisted.

I was longing to tell Mum, Dad and Ross the details. Jacques's parents and Sonia were also in on the secret because they'd brought the ring from the jeweller in Johannesburg to give to Jacques at Christmas. Sonia had picked out three beautiful diamonds, which Jacques chose from, then she had delivered it to the jewellery designer to make into the ring Jacques wanted, which was based on one that I'd seen and loved a couple of years earlier. He'd actually had it on him during the GoPro moment, but he had decided to wait until we could be in our special place. He knew I'd love that.

The moment my family saw the grin on my face when we connected via Skype they knew Jacques must have proposed. 'You look pleased with yourself,' Dad said.

'Jacques has proposed!' I blurted, waving the fingers of my left hand in front of the webcam.

They'd known it would happen, but not when, and were thrilled for me. They'd met Jacques quite a few times; he'd been to England to stay with us five times and they'd got to know him – and to like him enormously. 'We couldn't ask for anyone better for you,' Mum said.

After the call I messaged a picture of the ring to my closest friend Abi. Back came a message: 'OMG, can't believe it!'

At the SPCA the next day Maloli was bemused. 'I thought he was already your husband,' he said. 'But if he is not, then I am very happy that he will be.'

Yasmin and Liz were full of questions about Jacques and the wedding – most of which I couldn't yet answer. Deciding where, when and how to marry would take us a while. But there was no rush. What mattered was that whatever we did, and wherever we lived in the future, we would be doing it together.

That morning Maloli and I pulled up to a house where the owners had reported that their dog was itchy. We stopped outside in a large stagnant puddle that smelled awful. I jumped from the car, over the water, and carefully climbed a little muddy slope up to the barbed-wire fence surrounding the house. A large woman dressed in a long patterned skirt and top with a scarf around her head ran out of the house.

'Let me help you, *sisi*,' she kindly offered. *Sisi* – 'sister' in Xhosa – was what I was being called by many friendly women I came to meet in the townships. She grabbed my hand and helped me through the fence, then extended her hand to Maloli to help.

'*Molo, bhuti*,' she greeted him, meaning 'hello, brother'.

'You must help me, *sisi*,' she pleaded. 'My dog, *eish*, he is in a bad way. *Eish*, he itches and scratches a lot. *Sisi*, I love my dog, but, *eish*, nothing works. I'm so sad for him. He is so itchy. I even got him flea shampoo. I have no money to feed me and my children, but I love this dog. Please help.'

I was touched, not many owners would go to that trouble for their dogs. At that moment a little dog of about six months old bounded out of the house, before stopping to scratch with almost frenzied intensity.

I bent down to look at this sweet black hound that was more legs than body. He had lost a lot of hair around his neck and face, and his ears were almost bald. His skin was thickened from the inflammation and oozing in some places where he had broken the skin with his scratching. I was pretty sure this dog had scabies, a type of mange caused by a mite called sarcoptes, which is rare in England but common in South Africa. The mite burrows deep into the skin, causing really intense itching.

I started the dog on the treatment for scabies plus anti-biotics, because I was sure there was a skin infection on top, wishing I had something I could give to reduce the itching. I insisted that the owner must arrange for Maloli to come back weekly to repeat the treatment until all the itching had stopped, and for several weeks after to make sure all the mites had been killed. She was very happy to agree, and as we slipped back down the muddy slope and leapt across the water into the car, she stood waving goodbye.

We pulled away from the house and turned a few corners and as we turned into a new street five minutes later, we were met by a wall of people blocking our way.

'What's going on?' I wondered.

Maloli rolled down the window. '*Bhuti*,' he called to a young man nearby, 'can we get through this road, or has something happened to block it?'

'Yo, *bhuti*, I don't think you'll make it.' He looked sad. 'A man left his girlfriend's house just over there, fell down in the road and died. Nobody knows why,' he informed us.

'Oh my word. That's awful!' I was shocked.

'Thanks, *bhuti*,' Maloli said and started turning the car around, but by then there were too many people around us, so he decided to stop for a few minutes and let the crowd pass. He explained that there is a lot of sickness in the townships, particularly AIDS and tuberculosis, and deaths are not uncommon, especially when high disease prevalence is mixed with a high crime rate. I suddenly felt life was very fragile.

At that moment there was a knock on the window. Maloli wound it down to greet a man in his thirties with a bright-looking German Shepherd cross-breed at his side.

'Molo,' he smiled at us, then spoke to Maloli in Xhosa. Maloli translated for me. The man was wondering if we were stopping to set up a clinic. His German Shepherd was a faithful guard dog to him and he wanted to make sure he was healthy, and asked if we had anything to give him to keep him on top form. I offered to check him over while we waited for the crowd to pass, and the dog did indeed look good. For once, I was looking at a dog with a good covering of flesh over his bones and a silky coat.

'He looks great, there's certainly nothing for me to treat here. I could give him a wormer, but he doesn't need anything else,' I said. The owner was pleased and I squirted some Panacur into the dog's mouth as he looked up at his owner as if to say, 'Why are you letting this girl do this to me?'

Soon the crowd passed and we moved on to the next house. A dog had been restless and vomited a couple of times in the last day. The owner said he had been stretching out quite regularly, too. As I checked him over I suspected he had pancreatitis, since the only thing I could find was a pain in the upper abdomen. Pancreatitis is an inflammation of the pancreas. Dogs often get it after eating fatty meals and it is really painful.

An increased number of fats trigger the pancreas to over-produce enzymes and then, because there are too many enzymes, the dog's body actually starts digesting the pancreas rather than the food in the intestine. Signs of a dog with pancreatitis are nausea and what is called a bowing posture: standing on its back legs but down on its front legs to relieve pain in the upper abdomen.

In England you can do a blood test but unfortunately I didn't have that option in the townships of South Africa. Treatment for pancreatitis is with anti-inflammatories, ideally with the dog on a drip to make sure it is really well hydrated, plus eliminating fatty foods from its diet and giving it lots of TLC. Sadly I could only give the anti-inflammatories and hope the dog would survive.

My final week with the SPCA was a busy one, and on my last day with them, Friday 13th February, Maloli and I worked non-stop. We were grateful when we got to the last case of the day but, as often happened, it turned into several cases. A group of men greeted us at the house we had been called to, which would have scared me when I first started at the SPCA, but now I had come to realise that people loved the SPCA and respected us because we were there to help.

'*Molo, bhuti. Molo*, doctor,' one of the men greeted us.

He led us to his four dogs, all tied up around the yard.

'I'd like you to look at all of these dogs, doctor,' he said to me.

The first was a dog with a white eye. As I crouched down to the small, spindly brown dog to take a closer look at his eye, he became submissive, flattened his ears and rolled over.

'Sorry, doctor, he's scared of you. He's never seen a person with white skin before,' he laughed, before picking up the dog and plonking him on his feet again, telling him he was being stupid.

I wished I had an ophthalmoscope to look into the eye properly, or even some stain to check whether the eye was damaged, but I had nothing. Luckily, he wasn't squinting, and there was no tearing. The white colouring to the eye looked a lot like old scarring, so I was pretty sure it was nothing to worry about. He could see a little out of that eye, and he could see fine out of the other one.

We moved on to the next dog. She had a small cut across the top of one of her back legs. The owner explained that he thought the dog had been stabbed. I wasn't too sure, as the wound wasn't deep and it wasn't a clean slash. It was more irregular, much more as if she had caught her leg on some barbed wire. I cleaned up her wound and gave her a shot of long-acting antibiotics. The other two dogs were generally healthy and bright, so I just checked them over and gave them a wormer.

Finally, one of the men asked if we could look at his uncle's calf. His uncle lived two houses away, so Maloli and I followed him, along with all the rest of the group. As we went around the back of his uncle's house, we peered through the front door to say hi, but he was sleeping in the heat of the day, so we decided to carry on and look at the calf, which was lying in the shade. The calf had diarrhoea and was a little dehydrated. The SPCA wasn't equipped with many farm-animal medicines – in fact, it wasn't equipped with many medicines at all – but we did have cow antibiotics and wormers, so we gave it both, explaining that while worms and bacteria are two common causes of diarrhoea in calves, other intestinal parasites or viruses could be causing it, so they needed to keep an eye on the calf, encourage it to eat and drink lots and keep it away from other calves until the diarrhoea cleared, or let us know if it wasn't improving.

We came back to the SPCA centre at the end of the day, as we did every day, tired. But I always cheered up when I saw the centre's three resident comedians – two donkeys called Donkey and Winkie and a goat, Bok. These three were always together and I'm sure that Bok thought he was a donkey. They roamed loose on the SPCA property and we often came back to find that the three of them had made their way into the office and were causing havoc.

'Donkey wandered off down the road today,' Yasmin said. 'And of course Winkie and Bok followed. He's such a bad influence on them.'

'The firemen at the fire station found them in among the fire engines,' Liz said. 'Can you imagine? If they got called out for a fire, those three probably wouldn't move out of the way for a fire engine. They're so stubborn! We had to go and fetch them with some food, even though they are acting as if they haven't been fed,' she added, nodding towards Bok, who was eating the neatly pruned flowers in the flower bed, and Winkie, who had his head in the back of the SPCA bakkie, where a bag of food had just been. I laughed, looking at them.

'I'm going to miss these three,' I said. 'And all of you, too.'

At that moment a large white wolf-like dog caught my eye.

'Who's that?' I asked.

'Oh, that dog was dropped off here earlier today. The owner didn't want it. Apparently she's a useless guard dog. She never barks and is too friendly. She should be easy to rehome,' Yasmin said.

I hoped that would be the case. The SPCA had very limited kennel space, so each dog could only be kept for a few months before Maloli had the tragic job of putting them to sleep. After a warm goodbye I was off home.

Three days later I was heading to Uganda to work for a month with World in Need. I was sad to say my goodbyes. Yasmin and Liz gave me big hugs, refusing to let me go, insisting that I come back to visit the second I returned to South Africa. I promised them that it wasn't going to be the last time I would see them. Maloli, coming from a very different culture, shook my hand and thanked me for all my help and for what I'd taught him. I had really enjoyed my time with the SPCA, and I learned an awful lot about how to work in less-than-ideal situations and how to adapt what I had with me to the situation.

The following day was Valentine's Day. I had planned my trip especially so that Jacques and I could spend it together – it would be the first time we had ever managed to be in the same place for the most romantic of all days and I couldn't wait.

But over dinner earlier that week I had asked Jacques if he had any plans for Saturday.

'I'm playing cricket all day,' he announced cheerfully.

'What? But it's Valentine's Day.'

'Yes, I know. Don't worry, I'll see you in the evening after the cricket. Or you can come and watch, and then we'll be together all day.'

I stared at him in disbelief, inwardly fuming. I couldn't believe that he hadn't taken in how important this day was to me. Was he really going to spend it playing cricket? I knew I was always going to have to share him with sport, but couldn't he give it a miss for just one day?

The afternoon before Valentine's Day, after I finished my last shift at the SPCA, Jacques took me to a private game reserve, close to where he lived, to stay in one of their lovely little chalets. We went on a game drive and a boat safari on the Kariega River and while I was still deeply annoyed, out of principle, I had to admit that he had made a big effort to spoil me.

In the morning I expected us to drive home so that he could get to the cricket, but after a delicious breakfast of fresh mango and papaya he told me he wasn't going to play cricket after all.

'You're more important than my cricket team,' he said, and I melted. I should have known he would come through for me. I knew it cost him – it was a truly generous thing to do – so when we got back home that afternoon, having spent the morning driving around the Addo National Park, I insisted he go to the pub to watch the rugby.

Two days later, early on the morning of 16th February, I packed my bags and flew to Uganda.

Jacques took me to the airport for my flight to Johannesburg, where I would transfer to a flight to Kampala. I held it together until he put his arms around me to say goodbye when, as always, I dissolved into tears. I wasn't going to see him again for several months, and it felt as though each time we parted I missed him more.

CHAPTER ELEVEN

The Thank-you Chicken

Crammed into the back of a tiny car, my luggage squeezed up against my legs and several pineapples stuffed on the shelf behind my head, I watched in horror as we careered wildly through the streets of Kampala.

There were six of us in the car: me, my host – the Reverend George Amoli – his sister and her baby, his friend and neighbour, Vincent, and Liz – a Canadian peace corps workers who was engaged to George's cousin. There was also a mountain of luggage and the prickly pineapples that George had leaped out of the car to buy and then stuffed into every remaining crevice. Every time we swerved they fell off the back shelf, scratching the back of my neck.

The car was Japanese, with all the labels in Japanese and a clock that returned to zero every time we stopped, so it was impossible to tell what time it was or how long we had been travelling for. Vincent was driving us the 200 miles to

Owiti, the village where I would be based, and as we wound through the streets of the capital I had never seen such terrifying traffic. There were no lanes on the roads and there appeared to be no speed limits either; cars and motorbikes simply overtook anywhere they chose and drove as fast as possible. It was complete chaos.

It was Tuesday morning and I had arrived in Uganda the previous evening. My flights, from Port Elizabeth to Johannesburg and then on to Kampala, had been nice and smooth, and as we flew over the vast stretch of blue that is Lake Victoria, the second-largest freshwater lake in the world, I could see fishermen out in their boats.

In Entebbe Airport I was hit by a wave of heat that shocked me. I had thought South Africa hot, but this was far hotter and more humid and I felt instantly sticky. I was due to be met by Reverend George, who would be my host, but before I could get through to arrivals I had to go with my fellow passengers through the Ebola checkpoint.

Ebola was the virus that was spreading like wildfire around several countries in West Africa. It had already killed many thousands of people and the authorities were desperately trying to contain it. No country wanted to allow someone in who might be carrying the virus, so those who had it were immediately isolated until they either recovered — which was unlikely — or died.

One of the signs of the disease was a raised temperature, and as I had a nasty stomach bug that had started on my last day in South Africa after I cooked us a rather elderly chicken for dinner, I was pretty sure mine was raised and was terrified that I'd be picked out and put into an isolation unit. I was hot and nauseous and I looked ill but, amazingly, after having my temperature taken and being asked a list of questions, I was told I was free to go.

I emerged into the arrivals hall wondering if I would be able to spot George. I needn't have worried; he bounced up to me, dressed in his black suit and dog-collar, with a big grin on his face and said, 'Jo Hardy? Very pleased to meet you.'

After pumping my hand for several seconds he led me out of the terminal towards the car park. As we walked a sheet of insects that looked like mosquitoes flew over us – I'd never seen so many. Despite the heat, I put on my jumper to avoid being bitten, conscious that malaria was extremely prevalent in Uganda.

Vincent was waiting for us with the car and, after the introductions, George insisted we pray for the success of our journey before they drove me to my hotel and dropped me off for the night, promising to be back early the next morning.

It was a relief to have a good shower – my last for a month – and to sit on my bed, bug-free under the mosquito net. I couldn't make any calls until I bought a local SIM card, so I settled down to watch *Friends* on my tablet, but I felt too nauseous to pay much attention. The stomach bug was making me feel awful. On top of which I was in a strange land, about to set out on an adventure I knew so little about and I was missing Jacques so much that it hurt.

I had wanted to come to Uganda to help and to be useful, and I tried to remember that and to feel cheerful and confident about the coming month, but at that moment what I actually felt was ill and tired, a bit scared and also homesick, but I wasn't sure if I was homesick for England or for Jacques.

The next morning I managed to eat a couple of slices of bread and jam at breakfast but my stomach still felt decidedly dodgy. Half an hour later George and Vincent picked me up with the car now filled to the brim with luggage and shopping and George's sister, Joyce, and her baby girl Tulita, who got into the back beside me. A few minutes later we stopped for Liz, who smiled hello and clambered in beside us.

We were on our way from Kampala, which is towards the south of the country on the shores of Lake Victoria, to Owiti, a rural community close to the city of Lira, in Northern-central Uganda. Our journey took us on a wide detour around Lake Kyoga, much smaller than Lake

Victoria but still covering several hundred square miles. I was amazed by how lush and green Uganda is in the south and how as we travelled north it became so much drier. Much of the country is at a high altitude, on a plateau surrounded by lakes and mountains, so there's a great deal of agricultural land planted with huge crops of sweet potatoes, plantains, cassava and maize, as well as coffee, tea, tobacco and cotton. Over three-quarters of the labour force in rural areas is employed in agriculture.

George explained to me that Owiti was where his family home was, but that his parish, which included several churches, was actually three hours' drive away. Much of his time was spent at his parish, but in honour of my visit he had taken a month off to spend in Owiti with me. I was touched.

George, who looked as if he was in his mid-thirties but must have been at least a decade older (because he said most of his children were in their late teens and early twenties), was a warm, kind man who was very excited to be bringing me to the community. I was to be his honoured guest and to stay in his home, which was the only brick house in the area. I felt very touched by his generosity.

I had been told the journey would take five hours, but it actually took eight. We had several stops, including one in Lira where I managed to buy a SIM card, and several at the homes of villagers in the community where George gave away the pineapples that had made their presence so uncomfortably felt on the journey. I felt humbled that George was giving to the poor, despite being poor himself.

When we arrived it took some time to get all of us as well as the luggage out of the car. Stiff, sore and tired, I was nonetheless excited to see where I would be spending the next month.

We had been driving for the past hour through a rural area of rough roads and mud huts, but we had stopped in front of a small brick house, built around a yard on three sides. George's wife Lucy, round-faced and smiling, came out to greet us, followed by Joshua, their youngest son, who looked about 10. Lucy, who came from the local Luo tribe, spoke very little English, but she smiled and nodded warmly, making it clear that I was welcome.

George explained that he and Lucy had seven children. The two eldest, a boy and a girl, had died in a car accident five years earlier. Their daughter had been ill with malaria and their son was taking her to hospital when they were killed on one of the country's treacherous roads. It must have been the most devastating loss, but George spoke of it calmly. Of their remaining five children only Joshua was at home; the other four were away at secondary school and as there was no school locally they had to board and come home at weekends. There was also Kochas, a young man I gathered was from a troubled background whom George had brought into the household. George told me that he and Lucy also had several adopted children. If someone needed help or a home, he said, he would do his best to take them in.

He escorted me proudly to the newly built guest room that stood on one side of the yard. Painted green, orange and pink, it was a little room containing a very small bed and a small bathroom, which was basically a hole-in-the-ground toilet and a shower served by a gravity tank, which, he assured me, someone would climb up to fill every day. The electricity was provided by small solar panels, which, he said proudly, would provide light for about two hours each day, so I would be able to have the light on for a little while in the evening.

I was to be the first person ever to sleep in this guest accommodation and I could see how much trouble they had gone to. There was even a mosquito net over the bed, for which I was hugely grateful. Most Ugandans don't have a mosquito net; they are a luxury, despite the number of mosquitoes and the incidence of malaria. George told me he had built the room to bless his visitors, including those who came from World in Need to help. 'The more I bless my visitors the more blessings I receive from my visitors,' he said.

George was in charge of World in Need's operation in the north of Uganda. The charity aimed to help provide aid and education, mainly by donating funds to buy goats for the community – something that George was in charge of – and to sponsor children to go to school.

Supper that evening was eaten on our laps, sitting on bright blue plastic chairs in the yard. The food was cooked over an open fire in the cooking mud hut, which stood on the third side of the yard. Lucy had cooked a special welcome meal of goat, chicken and rice with savoury bananas and tomatoes. Joshua went round each of us, offering to pour water over our hands to wash them, and before we began to eat George asked me to say Grace, but by that time I was close to tears. I felt so touched by their generosity and the warmth of their welcome, which I didn't feel I deserved at all, and I was so tired and unwell that I felt suddenly overwhelmed and as I said Grace my voice cracked. With my stomach still queasy, I struggled to eat and soon after supper I excused myself and went to my room where I climbed into bed and, once I'd messaged my parents and Jacques to say I had arrived safely using the exceptionally slow and limited mobile network, sobbed myself to sleep.

The following morning, after a breakfast of a kind of flat bread, scrambled eggs and cold meat, George showed me around his small farm. They grew sesame and cassava as well as banana and mango trees and had a few cows and goats. When he was away at his parish, which was the majority of the time, Lucy and the children looked after the farm and were able to sell some of their produce and make a small income to add to the modest one he earned from his parish work. George also received a small payment from World in Need, but how he managed to support so many people on what he earned I couldn't imagine. School was not free, it cost around £60 a term per child and he was paying for his five and several others, too.

As we reached the goat pen George asked me to look at one of his goats, which had been mauled by some dogs. It was badly injured and although I flushed out the wound, sprayed it with antiseptic and gave the goat antibiotics, it died a few hours later. I'd come to the area to use my skills as a vet, so it didn't feel like the best start.

George showed me the five large boxes of medicines and equipment that the World Veterinary Service had donated and sent out ahead of me. David Shamiri of World in Need had visited a few weeks earlier and had brought out a suitcase containing all the goody bags the British Goat Society had sponsored. They had also helped with some of my travel costs, as had the Veterinary Christian Fellowship and the British Veterinary Association, which had donated books that I could sell to raise travel money. All these generous organisations had made my visit possible and I didn't want to let them down.

Most of the people of Owiti lived in mud houses with thatched roofs, scattered across a wide area around George's house, and that afternoon we set off on a walk to meet some members of the community. The first home we visited belonged to Anna, a woman in her thirties who was bedridden and dying of AIDS. Emaciated and clearly very ill, she managed to sit up in bed and she apologised to us for being so tired. Her daughter, Pasca, was out collecting wood, but I met her when she came home, a sweet, shy girl of around 12. Her father had already died of AIDS and she and Anna had no other relatives, no land and no animals. They survived, somehow, but when Anna died, Pasca would be alone. Before we left George gave them 6,000 Ugandan shillings, worth just over £1 and the equivalent of a day's salary to many people there.

Our next call was at Richard's house. He was a white-haired elder, respected as a highly placed member of the community. He welcomed me and insisted on giving me the money to buy myself a soda, or fizzy drink. I felt embarrassed taking his money, but it would have been rude to refuse, so I thanked him and promised to enjoy my soda.

A soda was a big treat in Owiti and when I saw the village water supply I understood why. The spring was situated at the bottom of a hill and the water that bubbled up from it, which was dammed into a pool with stones, instantly became muddy and dirty. People were scooping up water, using cups and bowls, and transferring it to big yellow jerry cans to carry home. At the same time there were several women washing clothes in it, animals walking through it and there was a steady stream of waste-filled water flowing into it down the hillside.

After meeting several more householders and gathering a group of excited children who followed us, chattering and laughing, as we walked, our next stop was a small tin shack that turned out to be the local Health Clinic. George introduced me to the friendly man working there, who was a member of his church. He was a public health worker, trained to take blood samples and run some tests in the lab, which was in Lira. It was hard to believe that in this tiny little shelter they were able to take sterile blood samples that could be tested for diseases like typhoid and malaria.

Near the health clinic were several other small tin shacks. This was the trading centre where people could buy a few basic provisions from men sitting on chairs behind tables, surrounded by goods in cardboard boxes. Quite a few of them were filled with sodas – Fanta and a sickly-sweet fizzy drink called Mirinda. The man behind the table politely brought out plastic chairs for shoppers to sit on outside the door while enjoying their drinks.

Uganda is a land of many languages, but most of the people in this area were Luo and I learned my first words: *apwoyo*, meaning 'hello, how are you?', and *apwoyo ber*, meaning 'good, thanks'. I would soon come to learn that *apwoyo* was a valuable word to know, as it could be used in many situations, not only as greetings – *apwoyo matek* meant 'thank you very much', and the usual response to that was also *apwoyo*, meaning 'you're welcome'.

By the time we got back to George's home it was dark. Uganda is on the equator, so the sun sets at the same time every night of the year, very fast, between 7.00pm and 7.15pm. After supper we sat outside and George told me about some of the local customs and traditions before wishing me a good night. I showered in water warmed to tepid by the sun and crawled under my mosquito net where I read by the light of a dim, flickering lamp until the electricity ran out.

I was keen to get to work, and the next morning George introduced me to the local animal health worker, Maurice, who was going to accompany me on all my rounds. Shorter than the average Ugandan man and very chatty, Maurice was about 25 and, like most of the men (apart from George, who always wore his black suit and dog-collar), he was dressed in shorts, a T-shirt and flip-flops made out of old tyres. He spoke good English and he told me that he had studied for a few years in an agricultural university. In most places in Uganda animal health workers like Maurice were substitutes for vets. He had little knowledge of farm animals, but he knew a bit about drugs and he was keen to learn more from me. I told him I wanted to learn from him, too, as he knew about the local animal diseases.

It seemed that Maurice had recently come out of prison. The story went that for some reason a neighbour came round in the middle of the night to the mud house where Maurice and his mother lived and their dog had bitten him. The neighbour wanted the dog to be put down but Maurice refused. The case went to court and Maurice was ordered to pay compensation to the neighbour. As he didn't have the money, he went to prison for six months instead. This seemed especially hard since the dog was simply doing the job it had been trained for. I was introduced to the dog in question – a small, black, shorthaired dog with a face like a collie – and she was lovely. She'd just had puppies, four little balls of fluff that I checked over. They were all healthy, which was good news, as Maurice was hoping to sell them.

Prison had interrupted his studies, so now he was studying alongside helping people with their animals in return for whatever payment they could manage; mostly some fruit, savoury bananas or cassava. But with limited knowledge and very little in the way of equipment, there was only so much he could do.

I had brought him a little box of health equipment: a stethoscope, thermometers, bandages, alcohol gel, syringes, antiseptics and extra gloves – and he was delighted.

There were about 120 households in the community, split into four groups – A, B, C and D. Each group had a leader and as George was considered the leader of the whole community, he had spoken to all four group leaders, two men and two women, explaining who I was and that all the groups would have regular visits from me.

I had piled a rucksack full of drugs and equipment such as syringes and hoof-trimmers to take with me that day, so Maurice and I set off straight away to work in group A, where I was based, visiting each home to ask if they needed help with their animals. Many homes had animals that weren't producing or growing as well as they should, usually because they were either sick or malnourished, so we treated the animals and also tried to educate the owners in how to look after their animals better.

We started with some cattle. I saw a cow with metritis – an infection of the uterus – another with diarrhoea and a calf with heartwater, a tick-borne disease that can affect farm animals of any age but is often seen in young animals. The calf had been spotted coughing for the past few days, it wasn't suckling very often and it was having mild tremors. Maurice recognised the symptoms; heartwater is unknown in England but common in sub-Saharan Africa. In the later stages the animal will die, but this calf was still in the early stages and I was able to give it antibiotics and tell the owner that it should recover.

By midday everyone had taken their cattle out to graze, so we decided that the next morning Maurice and I should set out at dawn so that we could see as many animals as possible.

After that, every morning Maurice and I set out on our rounds at 5am or 6am. We would meet each group leader first and they would show us who we needed to see. We covered those within a radius of a mile or so on foot, and for those that were further away we cycled. Maurice had a bike and George lent me his spare bike, which had a flat tyre and no brakes. On the slopes it was terrifying. I was constantly shouting, 'I can't stop!' as I rattled down the hill behind Maurice.

One day I pushed off my bike on uneven ground down a slope and, since there were no brakes, crashed straight into a tree. Everyone was laughing at me as I got to my feet, brushed myself down and said, 'I can cycle, honestly!'

One of the charities I'd contacted before my trip, the Worldwide Veterinary Service, had sent out several boxes of medicine and equipment in advance of my visit, so I had plenty of basic antibiotics, pain relief and so on, which was a great help because almost every household had animals with problems. With some of the extra money that had been donated to me by the British Goat Society I bought dewormers, too.

I saw cows, goats, pigs and dogs. All the pigs had lice, most of the puppies had worms and some of the cows were sunburned, as photosensitisation of the white patches was common from eating plants that they simply shouldn't have been eating. I treated a coughing pig that had, I hoped, just a bacterial infection, and two dogs with mange. Many of the animals I didn't get to see again, except the pig, whose cough I could regularly assess as the owners let it run loose in the day and it was often on George's land.

As in South Africa, people would say, 'My animal is sick,' and I would need to question them to find out what was wrong: 'Is it eating and drinking?', 'Has it got diarrhoea?', 'Was it like this last year or is it something new?'

A lot of people said their cows had no appetite, but it was difficult to assess whether that was due to illness or the intense heat. Several had East Coast Fever (ECF), another potentially fatal tick-borne protozoal infection in which cows have a really high fever and swollen lymph nodes followed by a cough and weight loss. At first when I saw these cows I wasn't sure of the diagnosis, because I'd never seen it before, but Maurice would confirm that it was ECF. All we had available to us to try to treat it was an antibiotic that was good against tough tick-borne diseases, although we knew that it was likely to be only 50 per cent effective. I felt frustrated that I didn't have the range of treatments to hand that I did in English practices, and I knew that I wasn't going to be successful in every single case, but Maurice assured me that doing something was better than nothing. At least we were giving the owners some hope.

By midday we would have been working for six or seven hours and I'd go back to George's, where Lucy had prepared lunch of rice, bananas and leftover meat. From the start I had a lot of difficulty with the food in Uganda because my system was not used to the conditions and the way in which it was prepared. The meat especially was unappetising and tough to start with, and once cooked it was kept in the food hut – there was no fridge – and used for each meal until it was gone. Between that and the muddy water used for cooking, I had an almost constant bad stomach and violent cramps. I began to wish I'd said I was vegetarian, because the fruit and vegetables were really good. But as meat was considered a luxury I knew it would be rude not to eat it, so I persevered.

Everywhere I went the people were welcoming. One of the biggest households I visited was run by a lovely old lady named Kijai, which Maurice told me meant 'first girl born in a family'. Kijai's house was a rectangular building made of mud that was home to several adults and young children. Kijai, who was the grandmother, came to me and knelt down, offering me her hand to shake. I was gradually becoming less surprised by this welcome, as it was the custom in the Luo culture for women to greet men and visitors like this. She led me outside to where five or six goats were tethered in a yard with a small shelter in the corner, built of wooden poles with twigs across the top and, in with the twigs, a tennis racquet.

All the goats needed deworming and their feet needed trimming. I did one and showed Kijai how to do the others, watching her and teaching her as she had a go, laughing with delight at learning a new skill. She asked me to look at her dog afterwards, but it was cowering and snarling, as if it was terrified. Several men ran after it for about 10 minutes until one pinned it down by almost smothering the front end and wrapping his arms really tightly around it so that it couldn't run away. I just injected in whatever skin I could get from as far away as I could with Ivermectin, the drug of choice in many African countries for treating and preventing mange and worms. I checked over the dog's two puppies as well; they were gorgeous, but had big wormy bellies, so they also got a jab.

Finally we went to look at the family's four cows. I was already discovering that all the cows in the district were wild and they could kick. The only way to examine them was to tie them between two trees, with a rope around their necks and another around the back leg on the side where I was working, which meant that sometimes the poor cows fell over. Two of these cows had diarrhoea, so I wormed them all and one more that I suspected had anaplasmosis, a little protozoa parasite transmitted by ticks through their saliva. With this disease the cow just looks depressed, apathetic and thin, so it's not always easy to diagnose. Occasionally, when it's really bad, the cow looks jaundiced due to the breakdown of red blood cells and the eyes look yellow. I had plenty of oxytetracycline with me, as it was the one antibiotic that would penetrate cells and treat an intracellular pathogen like anaplasmosis. After a long-acting injection of this drug the cow starts to pick up and makes a good recovery, so I was able to give hope to Kijai that her cows would get better.

As we left, Kijai, smiling and nodding, handed me a rather startled-looking chicken.

'It is to say thank you,' Maurice said.

I felt so bad taking one of the family's precious chickens, but I knew I couldn't refuse as it would appear rude, so I thanked her warmly and Maurice took a photograph as I held the chicken in my arms, the family all crowding round and the children squeezing and shoving to make sure they were included.

As we walked back I thought, This is amazing, my first ever chicken! I would have liked to take it home because Dad always wanted chickens, but as that wasn't an option I took it back to Lucy and gave it to her, and she promptly wrung its neck and cooked it for supper. Sorry as I was about my chicken, it was the freshest meat I'd tasted in days and as I tucked in I silently thanked Kijai. I was already discovering that the Ugandan people, despite having so little, were incredibly generous. Wherever I went I saw that people's doors were always open and, no matter how poor they were, what they had they would share.

CHAPTER TWELVE

Margaret the Pig

Not many of the animals we met in Uganda had names, but for some reason the pigs did. And Margaret was an impressive pig.

Felix was a young man who was a relative of the woman who led group C, and when Maurice and I visited the group it was Felix who showed us round. Before starting the rest of our visits we went to his home and met the fully-grown 200-kilo sow he had named Margaret. Pigs, along with cows, were the most valued animals in the community – cows for their milk and pigs to breed piglets, which could be sold. Goats were next in the pecking order, kept for breeding, for milk and for meat.

Felix was having trouble with Margaret because she kept digging up all his crops, so to solve the problem he had put a homemade nose-ring on her. This was something quite a few people had done with their pigs – sticking a piece of wire in through the top of the nose, out of one nostril, in the other, then out the top again, where the two ends of the wire were twisted together. With a nose-ring like this in place it hurt the pig if it tried to dig. The problem was that in most cases the wire was old, dirty and rusty so, unsurprisingly, it caused an infection in the pig's nose.

In Margaret's case it could have been a lot worse, there was just a small amount of crustiness from some dried discharge and the skin was a bit pink. I wanted to give it a clean and spray some antiseptic on it, but Margaret was not having it. The moment I tried to gently take hold of her nose she began squealing at the top of her lungs and charged through the crowd of onlookers – there was almost always a crowd wherever I went – heading off up the road.

Several men took off after her and eventually they managed to catch her and bring her, still protesting, back home. As there was no pen and nothing to tie her to, the men had to hold her while I treated her, by sitting on her back and holding onto her by the base of the ears. I was beginning to think it was going well, but Margaret had clearly been lulling us into a false sense of security because a moment later she shoved her very large bulk forward, knocked me flying and took off up the road again, galloping surprisingly fast for such a big pig.

By this time the residents of half the households in the area had come to take a look, most either standing around watching, or joining in the chase. A few minutes later Margaret was reluctantly returned, squealing loudly enough to alert everyone in the local area to her plight. With twice as many people hanging onto her and a lot of laughter from the rapidly growing audience, I managed to finish the job of cleaning her nose.

Poor Margaret. I would have liked to ask Felix to take the nose ring out, but I knew that his crops were too important to him, so we came to an agreement that if it started to look infected again he would get rid of it.

Leaving a rather disgruntled but hopefully more comfortable Margaret to rest under a tree, Felix took me next to the house of a woman named Afiya. She had two pigs named Katie and Engamagod (or so it sounded), which I was told meant 'trust in God'. Katie had just given birth to 12 healthy piglets – a huge litter in Uganda. Pigs can have up to 14 piglets in a litter, but in hot conditions there are often more like four to eight and some are likely to die soon after birth.

Afiya also had two cows, called Okello and Caroline. They were brother and sister and Afiya wanted my advice as they kept trying to mate with one another. I told her not to let them as any faults in related parents would be high-

lighted in their offspring and neither cow looked particularly strong or healthy. They were typical of the small,
hardy cows in the area and I imagined a lot of interbreed-
ing went on, since all the cows were free-roaming during
the day and only tied up at the homesteads at night. It's
always better not to mate two cows so directly related,
though.

Like so many others in the community, Afiya was touch-
ingly generous. I had done very little – treating her pigs for
lice and advising on how to improve Caroline's milk
production – but she insisted I leave with a chicken and a
large bag of nuts. Not wanting to hang a live chicken upside
down from the handlebars of my bike, as many Ugandans
did, I wrapped the chicken's wings in vet-wrap bandage so
it couldn't flap and placed it on the rack on the back of my
bicycle.

One morning, after a long, hot walk, Maurice and I
reached one of the final houses of the day. The heat was
scorching and I was tired from walking so far, so I was
looking forward to the afternoon rest. Sometimes I found
it hard that everything stopped for several hours in the
afternoon – life in Uganda was not fast and I wasn't used
to slowing down so much – but that day I was looking
forward to cooling my hot, tired feet while I watched the
chickens that played on the front step outside my room.

We had come to the house of a widow; a wonderful large lady with a big smile on her face who told us her name was Omondi, meaning 'born at dawn'. She was kind and welcoming and she told us that since her husband had died, her animals were her family. She had a dozen goats, several cows and a calf. I started by checking her goats. Most were healthy, they just needed worming, but the last one I looked at had a big bony mass on one of its back legs and the poor goat couldn't put any weight on it at all.

I wished I had an X-ray so that I could differentiate between a bone tumour, a callus around a break and osteomyelitis, but I couldn't, so I did what I could and gave a decent penetrating antibiotic and some pain relief, advising her that if there was no improvement the goat should be slaughtered.

We moved on to Omondi's gorgeous little calf that had been orphaned. The cow had died so the calf was now drinking water instead of its mother's milk and was being given food that its immature digestive system couldn't handle. I gave Omondi a rubber teat and taught her how to bottle-feed the calf with milk. This posed a problem for Omondi, because since the mother had died she had no lactating cow and so she would have to buy milk from a neighbour, but if she did that she would not have the money to feed herself. She was faced with the choice of going without food or watching the calf die. I felt so sad for her.

The following day Maurice and I cycled to group D, which was the furthest of the group areas and so too far to get to on foot. The group leader was a wonderful woman named Leonie, who must have been in her sixties. She was exceptionally resilient and wouldn't let her ill health get the better of her. She explained to me in broken English that she was HIV positive, very arthritic, and wasn't at all well. She had good days and bad, but no matter how she felt, she absolutely insisted that she was coming with us. Maurice got her to ride on the back of his bicycle so that at least she didn't have to walk.

The first family I saw had a litter of eight very new puppies in a washing-up bowl, along with a bony and very scared dog. They said the dog was the puppies' mother but I really wasn't convinced, as she didn't pay any attention to the puppies and she appeared to have no milk. I hoped that the real mother was in the vicinity because the puppies needed her.

As soon as I had given it a wormer the dog ran off, so I turned my attention to the puppies. I checked them all over, and they all looked well – full of life and bounce. They had obviously been feeding well from something. I wormed them all before the owner took them back to his hut and came back with some eggs to thank me before we hopped on our bicycles, waved goodbye and cycled away down the bumpy path.

Most households I visited had at least a couple of goats and a couple of cows, but the very poorest didn't even have that. One lovely young couple I visited had only five chickens and a rooster. Susan and Michael were probably in their late twenties and, despite having so little, they smiled warmly and made me welcome. They were worried about their chickens and explained that in the rainy season, when the crops were growing, they brought their chickens inside and the chickens would get 'coughs'. Since they were outside at the moment, though, and all looking healthy, there wasn't much I could do except give them advice on housing to ensure they had proper ventilation. Hopefully that would curb the problem next time. I also talked to them about the diseases that chickens routinely get and that are easily prevented, mentioning in particular that birds can get a parasite of the intestine called coccidia, and I gave them a medicine that could prevent it or treat it. They were so pleased that they insisted on giving me one of their chickens. I would have loved to say no, but that would have caused deep offence, so I took the chicken, hoping very much that this young couple would soon have one of the World in Need goats when a new batch was donated.

My next visit was to a family that was not much better off; they had just a few chickens and a cow. All the cows were tethered to trees at night, either by their necks, horns or leg, but one had tried to escape several months earlier. The owner explained that the rope had cut through the cow's leg one night just above the hoof, and the cow had lost her whole foot. I was shocked. I couldn't imagine how she was getting by without a hoof, despite the owner insisting the open wound had healed. But I had underestimated the cow. She was managing to get about pretty nimbly on three feet and a stump and wasn't easy to get hold of. Maurice and I tried herding her into smaller areas but it turned out she was still able to run very quickly through small spaces, and so half an hour later we agreed that we were wasting our time. She was clearly coping very well, and I couldn't see any obvious wound, so we agreed to move on to the next house before the day got too hot and the animals were led out to grazing.

The next morning was Saturday and George had arranged for me to give a lecture to the community on trimming goats' hooves, at which I planned to hand out the goat goody bags that I had put together before I left England. People started to gather outside George's house early on and soon there were more than 100 sitting on the ground in the shade of a large mango tree.

I had been told that after my talk and the giving out of the bags, people would celebrate, and I could see that many of the women had lit small fires and were cooking food. It was going to be an event, and I was the main attraction. I suddenly felt very nervous.

George was going to translate for me, but just before we were due to start he was called away to help a friend take his mother to hospital. He was one of the few people with a car in the region, and the taxi system in Uganda (large motorcycles called bodabodas) wasn't suitable for an elderly woman in ill health. He didn't return for an hour and in the meantime a lot of people decided to go ahead and eat. They sat on the ground eating, chatting and not in the least worried about the delay, while I got more and more edgy about my looming talk.

Eventually George returned and we began. To start with I was absolutely terrified, and very grateful that George was standing next to me. But after a few minutes I relaxed into it because my audience was so attentive and interested.

I had prepared a leaflet, with pictures, that I went through with them. At first they found it really funny that I wanted to teach them how to trim the feet of their goats, but when I told them what would happen if they didn't, they were shocked.

I explained that hooves continue to grow, and that over-grown hooves make it difficult for the goat to walk. Eventually their feet would become deformed and many goats become crippled. I showed them some pictures of badly deformed goats' feet and then showed them how to use the hoof-trimmer in the goody bag. I told them I would teach them to do this themselves, so that they could look after their goats.

I pointed out that some of the hooves I had already seen were wildly overgrown, so much so that I could hardly find the tip of the goat's toe and in at least one case I had actually broken the trimmer and had to use a second one.

My audience was rapt, they laughed at my jokes, gasped at the pictures of deformed hooves and showed great enthusiasm for learning how to trim their goats' hooves. Someone had brought along a goat, so I demonstrated the use of the trimmer. I also talked to them about general care, neonatal care, how to look after kids, what to look out for if the goat was sick and a bit about worms. When I had finished and had invited questions, a lot of hands shot up. I answered them one at a time and finally, an hour later, it was time to hand out the goody bags. The group leaders told them to line up in their groups and I gave the bags to the leaders, who then handed them out.

I'd ended up putting the bags together in the World in Need office the day before I flew out to South Africa in December and David Shamiri, the head of WIN, had brought them out on a trip he'd made while I was in South Africa. They were just little white carrier bags and in each one I'd put a copy of the booklet, plus basic equipment such as a rubber teat, the hoof-trimmers, rubber gloves and a calendar and pencils so they could circle the date when they needed to worm their goats or trim their feet.

I explained that it was important they use rubber gloves when handling goats' bodily fluids – especially after-birth – as the bacteria brucella is common in Uganda. It is a bacteria that may well not manifest clinically or obviously in the goat, but that transmits to humans and results in undulating fever – one with highs and lows that is hard to get rid of – and can affect the reproductive organs and cause miscarriages in pregnant women.

When the bags had been distributed people came up and thanked me warmly, and the feasting afterwards went on for some time.

That night, happy with the way it had gone, I slept well, until I was woken at 3.00am by someone playing 'Hark the Herald Angels Sing' unbelievably loudly. A Christmas carol in February seemed strange enough, but in the middle of the night?

In the morning I asked George about it, half wondering if I'd imagined it. He told me that a local man had died a few days earlier, when he crashed his motorbike into a cow that was standing in the middle of the unlit road. The way that people mourned was by playing loud music – African music as well as the carols – all night long, on festival-strength speakers which they hired, for a week. He explained that many African songs were deeply meaningful in their lyrics and helped people deal with their lives.

I felt desperately sorry for the man's family, but also rather worried that I might not be getting much sleep for the next week. I got used to it, though, and a lot of the music was African with a strong, deep beat. In the end I found it almost soothing.

There was little to do in the evenings but sit and talk, and I enjoyed walking, especially in the cool of the night. George, realising this, would invite me to walk with him, and we would talk as we walked. One evening, about two weeks into my stay, George told me his remarkable story. He had been born to a woman who wasn't married. She hated his father and didn't want her baby, so she instructed someone to go and throw George into the Nile. As this person carried the baby to the river, an aunt had stopped them and insisted that she would take George. But despite this kind offer, her family did not treat him well. They fed him and clothed him, but they didn't pay for him to go to school and they treated him like a slave. And when he had a bad infection under the skin of his feet they wouldn't take him to a doctor, so he had been left with deformed feet.

Knowing that he must manage alone, from the age of seven George started providing for himself. He wanted so badly to go to school that he picked wild fruit, sold it on the side of the road and used that money to pay his own school fees.

As he got older, he started planting some of his own crops and selling them. By the time he was around 13 years old he had saved enough money to buy a pig. He killed it, cooked it, and sold the cooked meat, which made him a lot more money and allowed him to become completely independent from his aunt's family.

One Sunday, his teacher at school wanted to go to church, but he was going to be late so he ordered George to take his seat in the service and save it for him so that when he arrived late he would have a seat. George had never been to a church before and he found it really interesting. When the teacher arrived to take his seat, George stayed on.

One day soon after, George became very ill. His aunt said she would take him to a witch doctor, but George was dragged there kicking and screaming and ran out, saying that the church had said he could be healed by Jesus. George recalled that as he broke away from the witch doctor's house someone in white greeted him, then everything went blank and he woke up on the ground with people peering at him. When he got up, he was completely healed of his sickness.

From that moment on he knew he wanted to work for the church, and gradually he made his way up the ranks of the Anglican Church, starting as a reader and then worship leader and finally a preacher. He got sponsorship through the church to go to Bible college and now he was not only leading his own church but was head of a large parish that incorporated about 40 others, and was highly regarded and honoured by a lot of people in the north of the country. When he lost his two eldest children in the car crash, even the President of Uganda paid his respects and made a donation to him to help with the funeral costs.

Having known such suffering and loneliness in his childhood, George grew up determined to help others and since he made that vow he has never stopped. I was fascinated by his story and filled with admiration for his courage and determination, even as a small boy, to survive against the odds.

I knew that paying all the school fees for his own children and several others was a struggle for him. He wanted to provide all of them with a chance in life, but it wasn't easy for him.

The school was built of brick, but it was still very basic. It had no glass in the windows, there were 60 children in each class, sharing the 30 desks, and there was no electricity or running water. But despite this the children were cheerful and well behaved. Some of them walked miles to get to school, but they went because, as everyone knew, education was the key to a better life.

I didn't get to know George's older children well, but I did spend time with Joshua and I really enjoyed talking to him. He was bright, kind and very caring, like his dad. He would walk several miles by himself to the local shops to bring back shopping for his mother.

Everyone I met in Uganda had a very strong faith. The two predominant faiths there are Christianity and Islam, although there are a few tribal faiths as well. When I accompanied George to the local Anglican church one Sunday, I asked him why there was so much belief in Uganda.

'In England you have everything you ever wanted or needed,' he replied. 'When you are in trouble you have the health-care system or financial help, so it takes a long time to get to the point where you feel the need to ask God for help. In Uganda the people have nothing and the only way to cope with life's hardships is to turn to God and their faith.'

The conversation left me thinking about how much I take for granted, the luxuries I have always had and not recognised as such, and how grateful I was for all that I have been given.

On another Sunday George asked me to take a look at a bull kept by one of the reverends at the church. It was a confusing system – there seemed to be four or five reverends and I wasn't at all sure how things worked at the church and who was actually in charge, but it all seemed to be perfectly amicable. One of these reverends had some cows that he kept at the church, along with a bull that had been tethered by its horns with a rope and was now injured.

I went to the land behind the church to have a look. The rope had cheese-wired its way deep into the bull's skull – the poor creature must have been in a lot of pain. I had to cut off the rope and it left an incision half an inch deep all the way around both horns. I cleaned the wound and sprayed it with antiseptic, then told the reverend to give the animal antibiotics for a few days and asked him if he could please find a kinder way to tether it.

Life was taken much more lightly in Uganda. It had to be, because death was everywhere. Everyone had lost family members in road accidents or to illnesses like HIV or cancer, conditions that often might have been helped had there been more medical funding and facilities.

One day George took me to the local hospital to see his cousin Sophie, who, in her late thirties, had terminal cervical cancer. I was shocked at how basic the hospital was. It was housed in several separate buildings, the surgical suite had plastic strips over the door and patients where wheeled from the outside straight into surgery. In Sophie's ward there were beds crowded down the sides and more in the middle of the room, end to end down the aisle. Some had two people to a bed. It reminded me of films showing hospitals in wartime, with casualties piled high.

In another part of the hospital George's sister's baby, Tulita, had been admitted with malaria. She was in a smaller room, with her mother and auntie, and to my relief they said that although she still had a fever she was doing well.

The nurse who looked after Sophie said that they had done everything they could and it was now in God's hands, an attitude which pleased George. A few days before I left Sophie was discharged into George's care. She was able to walk with aid, and sat under the tree cracking nuts with some of the other ladies. It seemed a much nicer way of spending her last days than being stuck in the overcrowded ward.

By the time I was in my third week I was used to the routine of life in Owiti. I enjoyed my early-morning starts with Maurice and had got to know many of the people in the community. Every now and then I went to say hello to Anna and Pasca. Anna grew weaker each day, and I worried about what would happen to Pasca when her mother died. Children in Africa have to be resilient and resourceful, but would she really be able to live alone, at just 12?

Richard, the elder I had met on my first day who had treated me to a soda, was also a friend, and it was at his house that I discovered what I came to think of as the ant-bite dance – something I became horribly familiar with during my four-week stay. I was worming one of his cows and, as usual, the cow was tied between two trees. Maurice was holding the rope around the back legs and I was trying to inject the cow, while the cow was trying to wriggle free. Suddenly I felt something stinging inside my clothing. I looked down and saw a trail of red ants making their way along the ground and … up my trouser leg. They had got as far as my top and they were biting me. Red-ant bites really sting and, as I might have mentioned earlier, I am not at all keen on ants, let alone when they're all over me.

For the next few minutes I jumped about, banged my legs with my hands, shook my T-shirt and twisted this way and that, all the while shrieking hysterically, 'Oh my good-ness, get them off me! Aaargh!'

When finally the ants were gone and I had calmed down enough to straighten my clothing and pick up the syringe I had dropped, I looked up to see Maurice standing the other side of the cow, a big grin on his face.

'I see you have discovered the ant-bite dance,' he said. 'Welcome to Africa.'

CHAPTER THIRTEEN

A Better Future

'We have got some very nice goats.'

George sounded pleased. He and Richard had been to the market in Lira to buy 34 new goats with the money donated by World in Need. They would be given to members of the community who hadn't yet received one as part of WIN's 'Give a Goat' project, but there were far more people hoping for a goat than there were goats to go around.

'How will you decide who gets one?' I asked George.

He looked grave. 'The community leaders have decided this.'

'Shouldn't the people who have no goats at all get one before those who already have a goat of their own?' I asked, thinking of Michael and Susan, the young couple with only a few chickens – one fewer since they'd given me one as a gift.

'No, we will have arguments then,' George said firmly. 'The leaders have said that every person who has not had a goat from World in Need, even if they already have a goat they have bought, may ask for one. And as there are many more people asking than there are goats, we will choose the winners from a hat.'

And that's how it was done. Each goat had a number painted on its side in pink, using some leftover paint from George's house, and then correspondingly numbered pieces of paper were put into a hat. Each person who was eligible would be able to pick out a piece of paper, and if they were lucky enough to pick a number between one and 34 they would get that numbered goat.

The evening before the lottery George asked me to check over the goats that he and Richard had bought.

'We got the finest goats in the market,' he said. 'But they are not all young healthy females, as we would wish. There are one or two I am not so sure about.'

In fact, he had done pretty well. Ideally the goats needed to be young females that hadn't yet had a kid, and there were quite a few of these. Some of the goats they'd bought were a bit older than we might have wished, but only three were actually sub-standard, and one of those had been injured when it fell off the back of the lorry as they drove home. It had dislocated its hip, which I managed to put back. I hoped with rest and pain relief it would be fine. Another had an infection of the jaw bone, known as lumpy jaw, and again I was able to treat the goat and was pretty sure it would recover, even if it was left with a malformed jaw. The third goat was the biggest problem; she was an old doe that might not have many years left to breed, which would mean she was of little use. At least she had milk streaming from her udder, a sign that she'd had a kid recently and so wasn't completely infertile yet. A few of the younger does needed worming, and then I was done. The goats were ready.

That night the goats were tethered to trees and Kochas agreed to sleep with them to make sure nobody stole them.

As people gathered for the giving out of the goats the next morning there was a real air of anticipation. Dozens of people had come to try their luck and it was thrilling to think that 34 of them would receive a gift that would make a real difference to their lives and to the wellbeing of their families.

Before we started George asked me to explain to everyone that the goats were of different ages and standards. I did, and I also told them how to tell how old their goat was once they got it, by looking at its teeth. It's really very simple; a goat is born with the potential for four pairs of incisors along the front bottom jaw. The upper jaw is just gum. They start off with growing baby incisors and every year they lose a pair and grow an adult pair. So if they have one pair of adult teeth and three pairs of baby ones, they are one year old. After the age of five the goat's age can only be estimated by looking at the amount of wear on the teeth, and as goats living on rough, coarse diets will wear their teeth away faster than goats on more refined diets, it was a bit of a hit-and-miss method.

As I demonstrated the process on one of the lottery goats, 50 people squatted around me, absolutely amazed that it was possible to tell that the goat was two years old. Behind them were 50 more people, peering over their shoulders.

By the time the draw was to take place, there were closer to 200 people. George held the hat and told everyone to pray as they drew their numbers because it was up to God who received a goat. They lined up and took out their piece of paper, and each time there was a winner there would be a whoop of joy.

Eventually there were 34 very happy people, each with a goat. To my delight, Susan was one of them. She had drawn a very good-looking, healthy young goat and she couldn't stop smiling. She and Michael led their goat over to me and told me their plan. They would sell the kids the goat would produce to buy cattle, then use the cattle to plough their small piece of land and use the money from the crops they could then grow to pay for their children to go to school. It was a perfect illustration of what a difference having a goat could make to a family. The first of their children, they told me, was on the way, so it couldn't have been better timing. As they were about to leave, Susan turned back. 'This goat will have a name,' she said. 'And the name is Jo Hardy.'

What could I say? Some people have stars named after them, some have goats. And personally, I prefer goats (but then I would, wouldn't I?). It would always make me smile, thinking that in Owiti my lasting legacy was a goat with my name.

The following day, George told me that he'd overheard some people at the trading centre saying that it was funny how all the people who got goats were those most in need of them, and four-fifths of them were those who didn't already have goats. It seemed the prayers had worked.

There was a second piece of wonderful news that arrived at the same time as the goats.

World in Need had also donated the money to dig a borehole to provide clean water for the community and, 10 days before I left, the work started. The man in charge of the whole operation, Bosco, good-humoured and outgoing, promised me that I would taste the water before I left. I didn't believe him; how on earth could a borehole be organised and drilled in 10 days when they hadn't even decided on a site?

The next day the surveyors arrived and located the best position – near rock on land belonging to George's neighbour. Rock means very clean water, so that was good news. The day after that the drill arrived and work began, with Bosco supervising the drilling team. The water was deep, they said, so they were going to have to drill a long way down. It was a tense wait to see if they could reach it.

While the drilling went on, I carried out my last few days of rounds with Maurice, visiting each of the groups with the aim of seeing everyone's animals before I left. The houses we had left were few and far between and the last couple of days were exhausting – we often cycled for an hour to reach a house on the outskirts of the community.

Two days before I was due to leave I heard that Anna had been taken to hospital. One afternoon I went to see her daughter, Pasca. I gave her a bracelet to let her know that I was thinking of her. I couldn't imagine being a girl of her age with no family at home and no money for food. The following day, Anna died. George paid for her coffin and friends came to help Pasca with the funeral.

I was deeply concerned about her. How could a 12-year-old, grieving for her mother, survive alone? George had told her that she would be welcome at his house any time and I knew he would do his best to help her, but his resources could only be stretched so far; I knew he couldn't pay for her to go to school and I couldn't help wondering what would become of her. George assured me that orphans in Uganda were common and the community would rally around her. Even so, I decided to talk to David Shamiri to ask what could be done to help her.

On my final day in Owiti the pump was fitted in the borehole and, true to his word, Bosco presented me with a cup of water. It was amazing – clear and clean and so good that it tasted just like bottled mineral water.

The borehole would make a huge difference to the lives of the community. There were excited, happy people crowding around the pump, desperate to have a go at pumping fresh water, some even drinking it directly from the tap. World in Need had also provided 130 new jerry cans for carrying the water, so that everyone would take home fresh water in a clean, new container. It was a world away from the muddy spring they were used to and would contribute to the wellbeing and the health of everyone.

On my last evening all the community leaders came to George's house to say goodbye. They brought gifts of bananas, eggs, nuts and two chickens. As, unfortunately, I wouldn't be allowed to take the produce – let alone the chickens – on the plane, once the leaders had left I gave all the gifts to George's family.

The following day I waved goodbye to George, Lucy and Joshua, and to Maurice, who came to see me off. I was excited about going home but sorry to say goodbye to my new friends, especially George, who was such a brave and warm-hearted man. His kindness had made a lasting impression on me, and so had the people of the community, with their resilience and generosity.

Before my flight home I had arranged to go on a tour for three days. I wanted to see a little more of Uganda before I left, so in Lira I joined three other travellers – Massimo, Pippa and Karina – and our tour guide, Rodney, on a trip to Murchison Falls National Park, three hours to the west. Massimo, in his late thirties, vibrant and spontaneous, had decided on impulse to fly from his home in Italy to Uganda, just to see the country. Pippa and Karina were sisters from Germany: Pippa was 18 and a gap-year student who had come out to work on a local project and Karina had come to join her for a two-week holiday. Pippa had been working as a community health worker in Jinja before heading to medical school the next year, taking blood from sick people to test for common infectious diseases such as malaria and typhoid. She had turned up in Uganda and received no training, so she had learned how to take blood from videos on YouTube and was soon one of the best at the centre. She would be miles ahead of her peers when she got to university the following year.

Murchison Falls is on the White Nile River, with the falls at the point where the Nile flows through a 23-foot gap to tumble 140 feet into Lake Albert at a rate of 11,000 cubic feet per second. The result is a dramatically powerful and spectacular waterfall set in a vast game reserve. We spent two nights and three days based in a campsite there, with no fencing, and late one night I heard Pippa and Karina whisper, 'Are you awake, Jo?' from their tent next door to mine. I was, and I could hear something moving about the campsite. We popped our heads out of the tents and saw several hippos wandering around. I held my breath – a distressed hippo can be very aggressive – but these ones were obviously used to being there and, with surprising finesse considering their bulk and weight, they managed not to crash into anything or trample on our tents.

During the day we went on game drives and at night we ate in the camp. The food was a joy. After four weeks of trying, unsuccessfully, to accustom my stomach to the food of Owiti I almost cried with pleasure when I was offered a simple cheese, tomato and avocado sandwich. I had missed fresh food – especially vegetables – so much.

Finally it was time to head home. I couldn't wait to get back to see my family. I settled into my seat on the plane thinking about how much I had to tell them, and promptly fell asleep. I was woken by turbulence as we flew over Sudan. There was a huge storm; I could see the lightning bolts hitting the ground. It was frightening and the lurching of the aircraft was stomach-churning, but eventually we made it through and I eased my vice-like grip on my armrests, although I was far too adrenalised to get back to sleep.

When finally I disembarked, 10 hours after I had first set off from Entebbe, I was tired, dishevelled and sore, but the sight of Mum and Dad waiting at the arrivals gate made me so happy that I forgot everything else. After hugs and tearful hellos, we had breakfast at the airport Carluccio's – the freshly squeezed orange juice and pain au chocolat tasted like heaven.

I had a week at home before going back to locum work, and it took me that long to get used to being back in the UK. After living in such basic conditions in Uganda I saw everything through fresh eyes. The fridge, the running water, electricity, the food and drink, my comfortable bed, our home, the car – it was a long list of things that seemed suddenly extraordinary. I realised that I'd always had everything I could want or need and I no longer took that for granted, because I knew that in Uganda most people would be amazed and grateful to have even a fraction of what we had. The experience of being there had been life-changing for me and I felt profoundly thankful for my life, and truly blessed.

Becoming engaged to Jacques had taken a back seat for the past month, since there had been very little time to think about it and no one to share the news with anyway. So when, a couple of days after I returned home, I went out for a family meal with my parents, Ross, and both sets of grandparents, it was lovely to share the news of my engagement and the story of the proposal with them. They were all so happy for me and Jacques, and excited at the prospect of a family wedding, too. They all toasted to the happiness of our future, and I felt a little sad that Jacques wasn't there celebrating with us.

I was longing to catch up with all my friends – it had been three and a half months since I'd seen any of them and it felt like an age. And of course I couldn't wait to show off my engagement ring and ask my closest friends to be my bridesmaids!

Top of the list was Abi, who I was hoping would be my maid of honour, then there was my fellow vet Lucy, my cousin Esme and family friend Becky. Jacques's sister Sonia was on the list, too – I'd already asked her in South Africa and she had said yes. I was going to need Sonia – not only was she brilliant with hair, nails and make-up, but she knew the groom pretty well and would help to keep us both calm as last-minute nerves set in.

I had bought some little rings which were knotted into the shape of a heart and in each little gift box I put a note saying, 'Will you help me tie the knot?' A little sentimental, I know, but I loved doing it and I wanted to give each of my bridesmaids something to tell them how important they were to me.

Abi and I got together for a girls' evening and when she opened the gift box she threw her arms around me.

'I'm so happy for you,' she said. 'You and Jacques were always meant to be. Of course I'll be your maid of honour. Er, what will I have to do?'

'Oh, everything,' I said, laughing at the look of horror on her face.

I saw Lucy a couple of days later when she came over with her dog Renly.

'What?!' she said. 'You're getting married and I haven't even met anyone yet. Honestly, couldn't you just slow down a bit?'

We went out for a long walk with our dogs Renly and Roxy afterwards and Lucy entertained me with stories of life as a farm vet. A couple of nights earlier she'd been called at four in the morning to help a cow that was calving. She'd found the poor exhausted cow up against a wall in the barn with the calf stuck because one leg was bent. The other was sticking out of the cow, but the bent leg needed to be straightened before the calf could be born. Lucy gave the cow an epidural to relax it, but had a real job getting the calf's leg straight because since the cow was against a wall she could only use her left arm, which, since she's right-handed and had always learned using that arm, was difficult. She wasn't sure she was strong enough but she managed it, before calling the farmer to help pull the calf out with calving ropes. It was a bit battered, and the cow was weak, but with a bit of TLC both survived and Lucy managed to get back to bed by 5.30 for an hour's sleep before getting up for work again.

We were so absorbed in our conversation that we hadn't noticed Roxy plunge into a very muddy stream. Renly was running up and down the bank, too scared to go in, so we gave him a push and he joined Roxy, although he didn't seem to enjoy it with quite the exuberance that she did. When they came out they were absolutely covered with smelly, swampy mud, so we took them back home and put them both in the bath, after which we had to change because they'd soaked us in water. After a cup of tea Lucy headed back home, promising to catch up again soon and keen to know what colour the bridesmaids dresses would be.

'I don't look good in pink,' she warned. 'Or yellow.'

'Absolutely no pink or yellow,' I promised, smiling. 'How about orange?'

She looked aghast.

'Only joking,' I said. 'The dresses will be elegant and tasteful, I promise.'

Esme was my 17-year-old cousin. She was like a little sister to me so of course I wanted her to be a bridesmaid. We had a family tea with her parents, Barry (Mum's brother) and Helen, the weekend after I got back and after the meal I slipped upstairs to see Esme in her room. I handed her the box with the ring and then when she opened it I asked her to be my bridesmaid. At that moment there was a throat-clearing noise from the computer and I realised that our private moment was being shared by the guy she was talking to on Skype! 'Oh, goodness, sorry,' I said.

'No, not at all, I was enjoying it,' he said.

Esme was the most amazing cook – she had made the whole dinner when we celebrated Dad's fiftieth birthday the previous year – so I asked her if she would make my wedding cake, too. She was excited by the challenge and said she'd get busy working on designs.

Becky was Ross's friend from university, and had become a close friend of mine, too. Ross and Becky spent a lot of time together during their time at university and after she graduated she became a special needs educator in Tunbridge Wells. She lived not far from us and often came to visit, and she fitted in so well that we soon came to think of her as one of the family, my parents referring to her as their adopted child. I asked her to be my bridesmaid when she next came to visit and she said she'd love to do it.

With my bridal entourage complete, it was time to start thinking about venues and, of course, dresses. Jacques and I had set the date for October 2016. That gave me just 18 months to plan the big day, and although it sounded like an age, everyone warned me that it really wasn't.

I missed Jacques so much. It had been difficult to contact him from Uganda, so we caught up over Skype once I was home. But talking to a screen was no substitute for a warm hug. He was coming to England in July, along with his parents, who were coming over to meet mine. Even so, three and a half months felt like a very long time to wait.

We still had so many decisions to make, including which country we would be living in after we were married, but whatever we decided, wherever we went, in 18 months' time we would be together, and that thought was so comforting in the long months when we were apart.

At least I had my horses to cheer me up. It was lovely spending time with Elli and Tammy, although when I first saw Tammy I was horrified! My thoroughbred looked more like a Shire horse. She'd had five months of rest because of her tendon injury and she was fat and fluffy. In fact, she was clinically obese. At least Elli had been exercised and she looked fine. I spent a lot of time in the days after I got back grooming, riding and just enjoying being with both of them. I trimmed Tammy's wildly overgrown mane and tail and put her on a diet to get her back into shape and looking good.

Thankfully now I could start riding her again, gently at first and gradually building up to longer rides. But after such a long break her dislike of being ridden was stronger than ever. She had plenty of tantrums, which usually involved bouncing around on the spot or, when she got very annoyed, rearing.

A few days after I got back I went into the World in Need offices to tell them how my visit went and show them some pictures. I talked to David Shamiri about Pasca and asked whether a sponsor could be found to pay for her schooling. At school she would not only receive an education, she would also be given a much-needed meal every day. Without the money to go to school, she would have to go out and work, or scavenge food from the land.

David promised to put her at the top of the list of children waiting for sponsors and a week later he called me to say that one had been found. Pasca had lost so much, but from then on her schooling would be guaranteed and that, I hoped, would be her passport to a better future.

CHAPTER FOURTEEN

Just Like Us

'Stanley is just not himself. He's picking at his food and he mopes around and doesn't want to play or go for walks.'

Stanley, a beautiful russet-coloured cocker spaniel, looked at me with sad eyes. His owner was Mrs Johnson, a tall, fair-haired woman in her forties.

'What's up then, Stanley?' I said, bending down to stroke his silky head. 'Let's take a look at you.'

I checked his temperature and heartbeat and looked him over for any signs of a wound, discomfort or infection, but he seemed fine.

Mrs Johnson looked worried. 'The thing is, we just lost his brother, Hector, six weeks ago and I really couldn't face losing Stanley, too.'

'What happened to Hector?' I asked.

'He had a blocked intestine. He was only eight. It seemed as though one minute he was fine and then three days later he was gone.'

'I think you've probably got the answer right there,' I said. 'Stanley may well be grieving. He's lost his companion. I can take bloods to make sure there's nothing else, but as there are no other clinical signs, I think there's a good chance that's the case.'

'Do dogs grieve?' Mrs Johnson asked, looking surprised at this. 'I had no idea.'

'Yes, they sometimes do,' I said. 'They can be very like us, feeling sad and a bit mopey when they have lost another dog or a person.'

'Oh poor Stanley, I didn't realise. I thought he was getting sick, too. What can I do to help him?'

'Just treat him normally; stick to his routine for food and walks and give him time. You can also get a collar or a spray that releases pheromones, the feel-good hormones, which can help to relax him. If you behave differently he will think there's something wrong.'

A relieved Mrs Johnson led Stanley out of the consulting room and I looked at my list to see who was next. It was my third day back at work, I had a full list of consults and most of them, it seemed, were Labradors. I had three booked in that morning.

Ten days after my return from Uganda I had started working as a locum at a village practice in East Sussex, a 40-minute drive from home. The surgery was in a single-storey building surrounded by a pretty garden, on the outskirts of the village. The front was painted bright yellow, so it was hard to miss, which was a real help the first time I had to find it.

The receptionist, Paula, greeted me warmly and sent me through to see head vet Joe, who seemed relieved to see me. 'We've been pretty busy,' he said. 'And as two of our vets are on maternity leave we're very understaffed. There's just me and two part-timers, Rita and Sue, at the moment, plus nurses Sammy and Kirsten, so I'll put you straight to work, if that's OK?'

It was fine by me, although it did feel strange to be back in an English practice again after months working in African townships and villages. I looked around at the shiny clean surfaces, sterile equipment, cupboards filled with the latest drugs and smart cages for overnight stays and the daily inpatients, and it all felt a little surreal.

Downe was a typical English village: a scattering of houses, a couple of pubs, a few shops and cafés and a doctor's surgery at the other end of the village from us. It was in a beautiful part of the country, surrounded by fields and rolling hills, and as it was early April there was blossom everywhere.

The practice was relaxed; Joe was dressed in jeans and a green scrub top and so was part-time vet Rita, who came in later on my first day and popped her head round the door to say hello. Over a coffee later she explained that she had two small children – hence the part-time hours – and so did Sue, the other part-timer. Joe had set up the practice with a partner, Tom, who had since left to move north after marrying a girl from York. Now Joe, himself newly married and with a baby on the way, was keeping it all afloat.

'With the number of babies all the staff are producing we ought to be setting up a nursery,' Rita joked.

'The practice is mostly small-animal,' Joe had told me. 'There are a lot of cats and dogs in this part of the world. But we get the occasional equine consult, too. I'll push those your way, if that's OK, as you've had some experience with horses.'

I was more than happy; cats, dogs and horses suited me fine. I looked at my list again. Labradors, it seemed, were especially popular in these parts. Fine by me, because Labradors are among the easiest dogs to treat. There's a reason why they're the most popular dogs, not just in Britain but in the world: they're well-behaved, good-natured, friendly, affectionate dogs, as well as intelligent and easy to train, which makes them great as working dogs or as family pets.

The first Lab to come in that afternoon was a gorgeous chocolate-brown chap called Hunter.

He was getting on – at nine he was an older dog and he was slowing down, sleeping more, and his owner, Mr Bailey, was worried that there might be something wrong.

'He suddenly seems very ancient and creaky, but surely nine is a bit young for that, isn't it?' he asked.

With good-natured, stoic dogs like Labradors it's hard to tell what's wrong. They don't tell you when or where it hurts by yelping or wriggling, they just stand there and look at you with big, sad eyes, just like Hunter was doing at that moment.

'I'll give him a general check-up and possibly take some X-rays. It sounds as though Hunter might have arthritis. It's common in older dogs and a lot of Labradors get it. Their hip or elbow joints are most affected and become inflamed and painful, which means the dog will move more stiffly and want to rest more.'

When I moved Hunter's back legs, he would look around at me as if to say, 'Please don't do that' – the closest a dog like him would get to saying, 'Ouch!' I kept him in for X-rays, as his owner was keen to find out exactly what was wrong, and later that day they confirmed the diagnosis, so I suggested a course of injections that would help to build up the cartilage in Hunter's joints: one a week for four weeks and then one a month for maintenance.

Mr Bailey's insurance would cover the injections so he was happy for me to go ahead, but he was less pleased with my second suggestion.

'Hunter is quite overweight, so you really do need to bring his weight down. The extra bulk he is carrying is putting an additional load onto his hips. Overweight dogs are far more likely to get arthritis than slim dogs.'

'Hunter isn't overweight,' Mr Bailey protested. 'He's got a little stouter with the years, but we all do, don't we?'

It was an awkward moment, since Mr Bailey was fairly stout himself, but for Hunter's sake I persisted.

'Well, no, dogs don't need to get any heavier as they get older and it's much better for them if they don't. I know Labradors love their food and seem constantly hungry, but it's better not to give in. Hunter really will feel a lot happier and his hips won't hurt so much if he loses a couple of kilos.'

Mr Bailey didn't look convinced, but he agreed to cut down Hunter's food by about 10 per cent and to come back in two weeks' time to weigh him again.

It's hard to change our habits, whether it's our own eating patterns or the way we feed our dogs. When you are used to giving your dog an extra treat, or a little bit of your leftovers, then to stop seems like depriving them. To make it easier I try to get owners to see that a slimmer dog will be fitter and live longer. Weight in dogs is a real issue. Of the four Labradors I saw that day, three were overweight. Unfortunately so few Labs are the right weight that some people think they're skinny and that the tubby dogs are the normal ones.

The next Lab to arrive was Jess, a young adult, in for her regular vaccinations. She was black, shiny and slender, but her owner, who introduced herself as Marnie, said that some people thought she was a bit underweight.

'No,' I said, perhaps a touch too ferociously. 'She's the right weight and anyone who says otherwise is wrong. Please ignore them, you're doing a great job with her.'

My last Lab of the day was Shadow, a glossy black dog of about seven. Her owner, Mr Shepherd, was concerned because she had a lump the size of a ping-pong ball just in front of her shoulder. I was worried; a lymph node swelling could be serious. I took a fine needle aspirate to get some cells from the lump to send off. Shadow had other ideas, though, and didn't appreciate me poking the needle into the lump. She wriggled straight out of Mr Shepherd's arms and hid behind him, panting. I made a second attempt, but Shadow wasn't having it and ran circles around her owner, tying him up with her lead, so I suggested I take her to get a nurse to hold her. As soon as she was away from Mr Shepherd she calmed down and was as good as gold while

I took the sample. It always amazes me how dogs pick up their owner's nervousness and calm down away from them, but of course the owners almost always believe the dog is happier with them. I took Shadow back to Mr Shepherd, praising her and giving her a little treat, and promised Mr Shepherd that we'd ring him when we had the result.

Sadly the result confirmed that it was a melanoma, a skin cancer that, in dogs as in people, generally has a fast rate of spread into other organs in the body. When Mr Shepherd came back in I explained to him that we couldn't remove the tumour, the site made it too complicated, and it would almost certainly have already spread. We could give Shadow steroids to slow the growth of the tumour and they would act as anti-inflammatories, too. That way she could carry on until such time as it was causing her too many problems. The other option was to refer her to an oncologist who could create a chemotherapy protocol for her, but understandably Mr Shepherd felt it wasn't fair to give Shadow chemotherapy when he wouldn't be able to explain to her why she was feeling so ill. I felt sad for them and assured Mr Shepherd I was always on the end of the phone if he was worried or had any more questions.

That evening after work I went to a gymnastics class. I'd started going regularly when I got back from Africa because I wanted to do something more than just work, go home, have dinner and go to bed. I was becoming aware that a vet's work-life balance is pretty precarious. The hours are long, the work is hard and it's all too easy to let work take over your life. I didn't want that to happen, so I was delighted when I found a gym class just a few minutes from home.

I used to do gymnastics when I was a child. I was really competitive and loved it, but when I was 11 I broke my arm doing a back flip and had to stop. Now, 14 years later, I had decided to give it another go and I was really enjoying it. The gym was international standard, training several next-generation potential Olympic champions, and watching them go through their paces was awe-inspiring. There was a great big tumble run with a foam pit at the end. I was practising forward somersaults, the idea being to land on your feet, with the foam pit there as a safety net. It was going quite well and I was, rather ambitiously, thinking of adding a half-twist to my somersault when, a few days later, Tammy put paid to my gymnastic hopes.

I was working her carefully through a three-month rehabilitation programme to strengthen her injured leg without over-taxing it. I had started trotting her in straight lines and every time we rounded for a turn I would bring her back to a walk, so that she wasn't putting extra strain on her leg. The trouble was, Tammy was having a stroppy day and didn't want to slow to a walk, so each time we turned and slowed down I had to pull tightly on the reins to get her to obey. After several tussles she decided she'd had enough. She planted her feet and reared up, then leaped forwards, wrenching my shoulder really hard.

I felt a jolt of intense pain and I was pretty sure, based on where the pain was, that I'd pulled the rotator cuff, which meant that there wasn't a lot I could do. Time would heal it, but for the next few weeks, and possibly months, it was going to be sore and gym would be out. I was really cross with Tammy. I loved her dearly, but sometimes our relationship was more love-hate than anything else.

The following day I went to the races with Becky. Lingfield Park racecourse is not far from home, and I had fond memories of spending a week working there with the vets when I was on my final-year rotations. Back then I had spent several evenings helping to check all the stunning thoroughbreds before the races and then leaping into a car with the vet to follow the race, roaring around the side of the track at breakneck speed, just in case there was an accident.

This time we were spectators, there for the fun of watching the horses fly around the track, marvelling at their grace and beauty and yelling for our favourites. I wasn't planning to bet, because I always go for the horse that looks like a sure-fire winner, nice and energetic with long legs, and then it loses. But before we left Mum gave me a tip:

'Pick an average-looking one,' she said. 'The one that looks like nothing special. They're the ones that win.'

I took her advice – I have no idea where it came from, as she has never bet on a horse – and won on every single race. Three of my choices came first and the other came second. I definitely owed Mum a box of chocolates.

Back at Downe the following week I had a day of equine consults, which turned out to be a lot of fun. I set off for the first call feeling a bit silly in my little car. I was pretty sure most owners and stables would expect an equine vet to turn up in a four-by-four, or at least a big saloon. Instead, they were getting me, in my modest but much-loved sporty silver hatchback.

My first stop was to see Chico, a gelding, for a vaccination. He was a beautiful chestnut horse and his owner, Mrs Grey, was a lively and energetic woman in her mid-sixties, but as I stood chatting to her, holding Chico's rein, he gave me a playful nip.

'Ah, sorry, I meant to warn you that he does that if you stand too close,' she said.

'Thanks,' I said, rubbing my arm. 'It's fine, he didn't hurt me, but I'll watch out in future.'

'Come in and have some tea and biscuits,' she invited. 'You must meet my dog, Perro. I've been training him and he loves showing off his tricks.'

I couldn't resist, and Perro didn't disappoint. A charming collie, he went happily into his routine: spinning in circles, begging on his back legs and, as a finale, shuffling himself, sitting his bottom on the floor, paws in the air, across to Mrs Grey, who urged him on with coos of delight.

'Oh good boy,' she said when he arrived at her knee. 'Isn't he doing well? It's such fun teaching him. We'll be on *Britain's Got Talent* next!' Then she roared with laughter.

After a cup of tea, during which Mrs Grey asked me, with real interest, all about my training, it was time to get going. My next stop was to see a horse that had gone lame at a stable a few miles in the opposite direction. The stable owner, Edward, took me through to see a pretty mare called Dixie. I started by checking her hooves with a hoof pincher, a tool which squeezes the top and bottom of the horse's foot. If the horse pulls away or twitches it indicates pain. Dixie seemed fine, so I felt all the way up her legs and watched her trot in a straight line on concrete. All fine so far, but when I did a flexion test, in which you bend each leg for a minute to stress the joint and then ask the owner to trot the horse, I could see obvious signs of lameness.

'I think her problem is in her right fetlock,' I told Edward. 'It's not dramatic enough to be a fracture or joint infection, but it could be arthritis, given her age, or possibly just a sprain. The choices are to see how she goes with pain relief and rest, or to refer her to an equine hospital for more tests.'

Edward opted for the pain relief and rest, promising to get in touch if Dixie didn't improve in a few weeks' time. As we walked through the stables on our way out, I started in surprise as I spotted one pony – and my heart leaped.

'Luna!' I said. 'That's Luna, I'd know her anywhere. She was my first pony.'

'Yes,' Edward said. 'That's Luna, she's a lovely little thing. Her owners keep her here and spoil her rotten. She's getting on a bit now, well over 20, but still very active.'

I went over and nuzzled Luna. I was sure she recognised me. My parents had bought her for me when I was 10 and I'd had her for two years. She was a lovely little jet-black cob with fluffy white feet and a long white blaze down her nose. It had been a huge act of generosity from my parents, but they could see how much I loved riding and I had begged non-stop for a horse of my own. And they felt that at least I would be doing something active and outdoors.

For two years I spent every afternoon after school at the stables with Luna, grooming and riding her. It was a wrench when we sold her to buy Elli, but I was ready for a bigger horse and we couldn't keep them both. Luna had gone to a lovely woman who had clearly looked after her beautifully.

Edward was right, at 22 Luna was getting on, but horses can live into their thirties and she looked a picture of health.

'I'm so happy to have seen her,' I said. 'It's lovely to know where she is and that she's doing so well.'

I was still smiling and thinking about Luna when I arrived at my last call of the morning.

'I'm impressed that you've got here on time,' the owner, Sally, said. 'Most vets seem to be at least half an hour late.'

'We do all try to be on time,' I said as Sally led me towards the stable. 'It's just that you can't always predict how long a call will take.'

Sally led her horse, a black stallion named Merry, out into the yard. I was there to vaccinate him, but he had some other health issues, too. 'He had arthritis diagnosed a few weeks ago and I've done very little riding with him since. He mooches around the field during the day, and at night I keep him stabled. He has a very easy life,' she said. 'But now he doesn't seem to want to lie down.'

Horses can sleep standing up, but they do need to lie down for a couple of hours each day to get a deeper level of sleep. Without that they become sleep-deprived. It's fairly common in old arthritic horses to see sleep deprivation, but it's very scary when you see it for the first time and you don't know what it is. If a horse is sleep-deprived and it falls asleep standing up, it often falls into a deep sleep, which causes them to rock dramatically and then fall over. Injuries such as grazes on the knees or fetlocks are a regular occurrence. I suggested to Sally that she give Merry a sachet of pain relief every day in the evening so that he felt comfortable enough to lie down to sleep. Also it would benefit him to be out in the field overnight instead of in a stable, as often older horses are not able to get up easily in confined spaces and, knowing this, they don't lie down.

As I left the stable to go to my car Sally nipped into the house and came out with a box of eggs.

'From our chickens,' she said. 'To say thanks for being on time.'

'Thanks,' I said. 'There's really no need.' But Sally insisted.

I'd really enjoyed my morning visits. It was lovely seeing Luna and I'd got a box of eggs as a bonus.

Back in the surgery, after a quick lunch, I was presented with a snuffly tortoise called Horace. He was only little, just six or seven years old, which is still a toddler in tortoise terms. They're the world's longest-living animals; most live to be at least 90 and it's not unusual to find tortoises well over 100 years old. Some have even made it past 150.

Horace's owners, a charming little boy named Ryan and his very nice mum, were worried that the tortoise was off his food. I explained that he had a cold. Tortoises have a very good sense of smell and, like most animals, when they lose their sense of smell they lose interest in food. There's just one antibiotic that's licensed for exotic animals and it's called Baytril. I told Ryan to put a little bit of the Baytril syrup on a piece of lettuce, or better still to inject it into his favourite strawberries, and hopefully he would soon be fine. With Horace back in his cardboard box, Ryan thanked me politely and carried his pet carefully out, his mum following with the bottle of syrup.

My last visitor that afternoon was Sonny, a lovely yellow Labrador. A friendly, smiley dog with a big waggy tail that never stopped. He was three years old, so still young, and his owners, a young couple who were as friendly as their dog, were worried because he'd had two seizures. They'd brought him in after the first one and had been told to wait and see if there was another. Vets never start epilepsy treatment after just one seizure because there are a lot of potential causes, such as low glucose levels or having something toxic in the blood, so it could be a one-off, but Sonny's blood tests at the time didn't reveal anything abnormal.

In Sonny's case, unfortunately, he'd had a second, longer seizure only a week later, so his owners, Becky and Jake, had brought him back. A second follow-up blood test showed that there were no glucose or electrolyte abnormalities in Sonny's blood and there was no history of contact with toxins. When that's the case, and the dog is between the ages of two and five, then the cause of multiple seizures is generally epilepsy.

Many people don't realise that dogs can get epilepsy. When a seizure is coming on the owner may notice the dog acting strangely, or seeming upset or nervous, repeating motions, hiding or demanding extra attention. At this stage, which can last for anything from a few minutes to a couple of hours, the seizure is beginning in one part of the brain. As it spreads to the whole brain the dog will go rigid, its legs straight out and head back, before starting to seize. It will lose consciousness and usually become doubly incontinent. Although its eyes may be open, it won't be seeing anything. This stage usually lasts no more than a minute or two, but for the owner it can be alarming to watch. After the seizure the dog will probably be rather quiet and behave strangely again for several hours to a day.

Luckily there are good medications for treating it. The medication won't cure the epilepsy, but in a lot of cases it will significantly reduce the number of seizures.

I explained all of this to Becky and Jake and did my best to put them at ease. Hopefully, I said, Sonny's epilepsy would be brought under control. I asked them to keep a diary of his seizures – how often they occurred and how long they went on for – and explained that it's not a good

idea to touch a dog having a seizure, as it may unintention-
ally bite. They should remove all furniture from around
him, though, and make sure they were timing the seizure,
and if it went on longer than two minutes they should rush
him to the vet. Once the pattern of Sonny's seizures was
established, I explained, we would be able to increase or
lower the medication and get it to the right level. There
was a fairly new drug that was having good results and was
very safe compared with older epilepsy medication, so
Sonny would be put on that to begin with.

'Will it be for the rest of his life?' Becky asked, her eyes
full of tears.

'I'm afraid it will,' I said. 'I know it's a shock, but you
will get used to managing it. He'll need tablets every day.
But just like many people with epilepsy, most dogs that
have it lead full and active lives.'

I couldn't help reflecting as I drove home that man's best
friend does share many of man's maladies. They may be on
four legs and be descended from wolves, but in so many
ways they are still just like us.

CHAPTER FIFTEEN

The Trouble with Cats

If dogs are pretty easy to read, cats can often be complete mysteries. Unlike dogs, they roam away from the home on their own in a world that is totally separate to ours, and most of the time we have no idea what they get up to.

Cats like to be independent. They don't need to be walked or taken outside, they prefer to patrol their territory and be their own bosses. They don't like too much interference or fussing. And they absolutely hate going to the vet.

An owner will arrive with their cat in a crate, open it up on the consulting-room table and, predictably, the cat refuses to come out.

'It took me ages to get her in there,' the puzzled owner will say. 'I just don't understand why she won't come out.'

Because she's at the vet's.

It's extraordinary how, despite the fact that there's nothing in the cat crate to hold onto, a cat can jam itself inside so firmly that it takes a lot of coaxing, prising and effort to get it out. At which point some cats give in, while others make their displeasure clear by biting or swiping at the hapless vet. Many dogs will patiently put up with a vet gently prodding and poking to find out what's wrong, and warn you by growling if they're thinking of snapping at you, but cats give no warning at all – then they can object, loudly and speedily, claws unleashed and sharp little teeth at the ready. The only indication of approaching trouble is the occasional twitch of the very tip of the tail.

Owners are always terribly embarrassed when their cats bite or scratch, but we tell them it's not their fault – the cat is in a strange environment and doesn't like it.

Don't get me wrong, I love cats, and I know that some are docile, easy to manage, cute little felines, but others, as every vet knows, are tigers hiding inside the bodies of apparently innocent moggies. Do something they don't like and suddenly it's war.

Cats get stressed very easily. A lot of feline complaints are due to stress, and one of the biggest causes is change, of any sort. Owners often don't realise that even something small – moving the furniture around, having strangers in the home, a new cat in the neighbourhood – can provoke stress symptoms in their cat. As for a major change, like moving home, many cats protest by simply disappearing for days at a time.

In my second week at Downe I had a run of cat cases that reminded me of just how hard cats can be to understand. One morning Joe asked me to go on a house call to see an elderly woman who wasn't able to bring her cat into the surgery. The cat had been diagnosed with cystitis the week before and it didn't seem to be clearing up. He suggested that, as I was new to the practice and the area, I take Sammy with me. Sammy was a cheerful, bright young nurse and she knew the way to Mrs Dixon's house, so I was glad of her company.

When we arrived Mrs Dixon, who was in her eighties, introduced us to her rather elderly ginger cat, Clarice, who glared at us from behind a chair.

'I've shut her cat flap so that she can't get out,' Mrs Dixon explained. 'But she's not happy about it.'

We could see that. Clarice may have been elderly, but she clearly had plenty of fight in her.

I asked Mrs Dixon how Clarice was doing.

'She's still using the litter tray, far more often than usual, and she seems to be agitated. She's had antibiotics, but it hasn't cleared up. Is there something else we can try?'

Cystitis, in other words an inflamed bladder, is common in cats. And while in dogs the cause may be a bacterial infection, cats have very concentrated urine that kills off bacteria, so the more common cause of their cystitis is stress. We call it Feline Idiopathic Cystitis – 'idiopathic' meaning of unknown cause. When that happens a bit of detective work is often what's needed.

'Has there been any change in Clarice's routine, or in your home, lately?' I asked.

'Well, no, I don't think so,' Mrs Dixon said, pausing to think. 'The only thing that's different is that I've had a new back door fitted. But it couldn't be that, could it?'

'May I have a look at it?' I asked.

The old lady led Sammy and I through to her small kitchen. There was the smart new door – with glass panels fitted in the top and bottom.

'Did the door have glass in it before?' I asked.

'Actually, it didn't. I wanted glass because the kitchen was so dark. It's much lighter now; I'm really pleased with it. That wouldn't be what's bothering Clarice, would it?'

'It could be. Has she been reacting to the new door in any way?'

'Now you come to mention it, there's a tomcat next door that sometimes hangs around outside, especially with this new door. He parades in front of it. Clarice doesn't like it at all. When she sees him there, she runs out of the room.'

'I think that might be the cause of her stress. Perhaps you could cover the glass in the bottom half of the door with cardboard and see how she is then. I'm sorry, it will mean a bit less light in the room, but you won't need to cover the top half, just the bit at Clarice's eye level. And if it makes a difference we have our answer.'

'Goodness, I would never have thought that could be a problem,' Mrs Dixon said. 'Poor Clarice, she must be feeling very upset.'

'If we've found the cause, she'll soon be better,' I said. 'And in the meantime make sure she gets as much water as possible, it will help ease the symptoms. Put a bit of water in her food and try running the cold tap slowly – cats love running water and she may drink from it. I'll give her some anti-inflammatories, too. Give me a call in a few days and let me know how she's doing. If she's not better we can run some more tests.'

It's always nice to do a bit of detective work and come up trumps, so I was really pleased when, five days later, Mrs Dixon rang to say that Clarice was much better.

Problem solved.

Another stress reaction in cats is pulling their hair out. When they're upset they often over-groom and they have such rough tongues that they create bald patches where they break the skin, which can lead to infections.

A day or two after visiting Mrs Dixon a tearful woman brought in her cat, Olive, a little tabby with a couple of nasty-looking bald patches on her belly and back legs.

'I don't know why she's doing this,' her owner, Mrs James, said. 'She sits on my lap licking at herself and I can't stop her.'

'Let's start with a few tests,' I said. 'We'll do our best to get to the bottom of it.'

After prising Olive reluctantly from her cat crate I gently checked her over, before taking a sample of blood and some skin samples, a few hairs and a tape impression of the bald patches (sticky tape pressed onto the skin to get some cells).

'We'll run some tests on this and I'll call you with the results,' I told Mrs James. 'But in the meantime see if anything at home or in her routine has changed. The problem may be stress, and if it is then she may want to feel safe by hiding. You can even feed her in a quiet corner where she feels hidden away and put litter trays in unusual sheltered places. It might help her feel more secure.'

The test results came back a day or two later clear of any medical cause for Olive's behaviour. I phoned Mrs James to let her know and to say that I'd leave out some cream for her to collect, to calm the redness on the worst of Olive's bald patches where her saliva had caused a mild skin infection.

Mrs James had been so upset when she came in, but over the phone she sounded a lot more cheerful.

'I think I know what's wrong with Olive,' she said. 'We've been having some work done in the house, a new bathroom, so the plumbers have been going in and out and making quite a bit of noise. I've been watching Olive and each time they come in she runs to hide behind a chair. As soon as I realised it might be that I made sure that Olive was nowhere near them and moved her bed and her feeding bowl to a quieter part of the house. She already seems a little better and as the plumbers will be finished tomorrow I'm hoping that will sort things out.'

I was very glad to hear it, and asked her to let me know how Olive was getting on.

While stresses in the home can be a problem, what cats get up to outside is often worse.

When cats go out at night, and many cats do, they get up to all sorts of mischief. Fights, falls, eating something poisonous and collisions with cars can all result in the cat coming home sick or injured and it can be difficult to know what the cause is.

Sophie was a pretty little white cat who was brought in by her owner because she had arrived home that morning with her back hunched, tip-toeing on her back legs and with a droopy, dragging tail.

The moment I touched her tail she yowled. It was clearly very painful and X-rays showed that there was damage in the sacral area of her lower spine. She had been injured, and the most likely cause was that her tail had been run over. Cats flee from the path of a car, and often it's their tail that doesn't quite make it. The result is a lot of pain for the poor cat and often the loss of bladder or bowel control – an injury called, appropriately, a tail-pull.

In many cases the cat's tail has to be amputated, and in the worst cases, when the cat can't regain bladder and bowel control, it has to be put to sleep. But I was hoping that Sophie would be one of the lucky ones. Her injury wasn't the most severe and she stood a 50/50 chance of recovering.

I gave her a pain-relief injection and told her worried owner that I wanted to keep her in for a day or two to monitor whether she had any control of her bowels and give her strong pain relief. After 24 hours I was convinced she could urinate and defecate with some degree of control, so I sent her home with strict instructions to keep her quiet and rested. It took several visits over the following weeks, but Sophie did make a steady recovery, including use of her tail again, much to her owner's relief.

My next visitor was Bob, an elderly black tomcat who had disappeared for a week and then reappeared with a large swelling on his face. His owner, a builder named Andy, a broad-shouldered, sturdy and cheerful man in his forties, was glad to have him back, but concerned about the state he was in.

He may have been getting on in years, but Bob was a proper tomcat. He had never been castrated and, like all un-neutered toms, his face had grown larger and he stank to high heaven. The swelling on his face was so large that his eye was almost shut. He had a temperature and his coat was dull and greasy.

'It's what we call a cat-bite abscess,' I told Andy. 'He's probably been fighting and had a bite or a scratch that has become infected and developed into an abscess. Luckily it's fairly easy to treat.'

A cat abscess is pretty common, and while they're not all a result of fighting, a lot of them are. Cats, especially male ones, do fight. It's a territorial thing; they like to guard their own little realm and an invader is not usually welcome. Sometimes owners get a second cat to keep the first one company and the result is disaster – the first cat may see the newcomer as a threat, not a pal. Cats are solitary characters.

I clipped the fur on the side of Bob's face, cleaned it with antiseptic and then stuck in a needle to make 100 per cent sure it was an abscess. Then, using a small scalpel, I made a little incision into the abscess to drain it – which took quite some time – before washing it out with antiseptic. Bob behaved beautifully and I was grateful to him, because draining an abscess is one of my least favourite jobs and an angry cat on top would not have helped. The procedure sounds as if it would hurt, but relief of the pressure actually far outweighs the pain of the incision.

I sent Andy home with pain relief and antibiotics for Bob and told him to wash the abscess twice a day with salt water and to keep the hole open so that it could continue to drain.

'In a few days,' I told him, 'Bob will be fine. And no doubt ready to go off on another jaunt, hunting and fighting. Won't you, Bob?'

But Bob was looking bored. His secret world was his alone. He was a chunky cat, and no doubt caught himself a few extra meals when he was out at night. It's something owners often don't take into account. Cats get fat and owners protest that they feed them the correct amounts. But cats often supplement their meals at home with tasty morsels like mice, voles and birds, and these extra snacks can sometimes be the source of problems as well as plenty of extra calories.

My next patient, Lily, was a pretty tabby brought in to

see me because she was vomiting and had tremors. Her owner had rushed her in after dropping the children at school.

'Lily keeps twitching,' she said. 'What on earth do you think has happened?'

As is so often the case with cats, I had to look at the available facts and guess. After a clinical exam, and a check on her sugar levels to make sure they weren't low, I was pretty sure that Lily had been poisoned, probably by something she'd eaten while out on the prowl.

'We'll need to keep her in,' I told Mrs Needham. 'I'll put her on a drip to try to flush anything toxic out of her system and we'll keep a close eye on her.'

'Can I bring the children to see her?' Mrs Needham asked. 'They adore her and they'll be worrying about her.'

'Yes, of course you can. It will be good for Lily to see you and the children. She's going to be in a cage in a strange place, and feeling unwell, too, so I'm sure a visit would do her good.'

That afternoon Mrs Needham arrived with Ben, ten and Chloe, eight. The children, still in their school uniforms, were very quiet, but as soon as they saw Lily they brightened. I opened the cage door so that they could stroke her and she lay quietly and purred.

After that the family came in every day to see her, and as Lily gradually improved they were full of excitement. By the time she was pronounced well enough to go home, three days later, Ben and Chloe were chattering happily and fighting over who would hold the cat crate and who would feed Lily when they got home.

'Thank you,' Mrs Needham said. 'Did you ever have any idea what had poisoned Lily?'

'No,' I said. 'There's really no way to tell. It could be any number of things: toads, slug pellets, toxic plants and some human foods are poisonous for cats. But she's a strong little cat and hopefully it won't happen again.'

I saw another little survivor the next day. Jazz, a lovely, soft grey cat, was rushed into the practice by her owner, Helen, after she was hit by a car. Unusually, Helen had actually seen the accident and she was beside herself. A pretty woman in her early thirties, with shoulder-length dark hair, I recognised her from the local bank where she worked. She arrived with Jazz in her arms and laid her on the consulting-room table. Jazz was conscious, wide-eyed and clearly very startled.

'The car hit her full on,' Helen said. 'I'd just got home and Jazz dashed out of the house. It wasn't the driver's fault, he didn't have a chance to see her and he was terribly sorry. Please tell me she's going to be all right.'

I reassured Helen that we would do our best and I asked Paula, the receptionist, to make her a cup of tea while I examined and X-rayed Jazz.

An hour later I went out to find Helen, who was sitting in the waiting room.

'Jazz hasn't got any major internal injury, which is great news. We worry about ruptured diaphragms or bladders or broken bones and she hasn't got any of those. But she has some nasty cuts on the inside of her back legs, and she has a lot of soft-tissue swelling around them.'

Helen gasped. 'Oh no. Will she be all right?'

'Yes, she should make a full recovery. She probably feels pretty miserable at the moment, but I've given her pain relief and cleaned the wounds with antiseptic. She should feel a little easier soon. You can take her home, but she's going to have trouble walking comfortably for a few days. She needs lots of TLC, and of course if you're at all worried bring her straight back in.'

Half an hour later Helen left with a very sleepy Jazz wrapped in her coat.

'Thank you,' she said, tears in her eyes. 'I thought I'd lost her. I don't know what I'd do without her.'

'She's lucky,' I said. 'Lucky to have survived and lucky to have an owner who cares so much and who got her straight to us.'

What happened to Jazz is all too common. Most veterinary practices get cats coming in every week with injuries that indicate they've been in an RTA – road traffic accident. One of the ways you can tell is that after an RTA if you press the cat's feet to get them to extend their claws they're often scuffed because they've been dragged along the road by the car with the cat trying to brace with its claws.

If the cat is lucky it will make a full recovery, but sometimes they're left with residual effects of their injuries that can be hard to live with – for the cat and for the owner.

Mary was devoted to her cat Jeremy. Her children had grown up and left home and her husband had died, so Jeremy, a quiet, good-natured cat with black-and-brown striped markings, was her only companion. The two of them got on very well, until one day Jeremy was hit by a car. His spine was damaged and as a result he had a lot of muscle wastage in his back legs. He couldn't jump and could only pull himself up onto a chair using his front legs.

Jeremy had been coming in every couple of weeks for check-ups, but he was making very slow progress. I suggested to Joe that I might be able to help out by teaching Mary some simple exercises she could do with Jeremy to help strengthen his back legs. While not trained as an animal physiotherapist – they are highly trained professionals who do a physio degree followed by a Masters in animal physio – I had picked up some useful tips during my neurological placement in my final year.

Joe was happy for me to go ahead, so I asked Mary to book in with a double-length appointment. She was delighted that there might be something she could do to help Jeremy, and she paid close attention as I showed her some massage techniques and something called 'passive range of motion' in which you gently pump the animal's legs up and down, flexing and extending. Essentially you move the leg for the animal, but it still means that the animal's muscles are working and growing stronger.

I also showed her a technique that helps the postural core muscles. You fill up a water bottle so that you have a wobbly surface and then put the animal's back legs on it. That helps the animal with posture, spatial awareness and core muscles.

Mary went away promising to work through the exercises with Jeremy several times a day and when I revisited Downe for a few locum days a month later she called to say that Jeremy's back-leg strength had improved.

It feels good to be able to do something positive, and as vets most of the time we can. But sometimes all our best efforts fail, and it's always the failures we remember most. Sweetie was a cat who stayed on my mind for a long time after I treated him.

He was a beautiful young black-and-white cat who was brought in by a whole family – mum, dad and three young children. They explained, all talking over one another, that Sweetie had suddenly been unable to use his back legs. One day he was fine, and the next morning he couldn't walk.

'What's wrong with him?' said the smallest girl, who must have been about six. 'Is he going to get better? I chose his name,' she added.

'I need to have a look at Sweetie and then I'll let you know,' I told her.

Actually, I thought I knew what was wrong, and it wasn't good. I checked Sweetie over. His back legs were stone cold and his temperature was low. All the signs pointed to an aortic thromboembolism. This is when a blood clot forms in the heart and then travels down to the fork of the blood vessels that supply the back legs and lodges there.

I explained to the family that we would need to keep Sweetie in our pet hospital to try to help him and promised to call them. They left, after kissing him goodbye, all of them looking sad and subdued.

I started Sweetie on strong pain relief every six hours and aspirin therapy in the hope of dissolving the blood clot, but I knew that the chances of him recovering were very low. Two days went by with no improvement and it was starting to become hard to manage his pain. He hadn't regained any function of his back legs and they were still very cold.

I phoned the family and spoke to Mr Barnes. As always, in these situations, I outlined what we had done and told him that the prognosis wasn't good and that Sweetie was in a lot of pain.

The decision always lies with the owner. We vets can only give them the facts, but most owners don't want their pet to suffer. Mr Barnes phoned me back to say that the family would like to say goodbye to Sweetie and then they wanted me to put him out of his pain.

They arrived an hour later and all three children were so brave. They took turns to cuddle their pet and kiss him goodbye. When it came to the smallest girl's turn she buried her blonde head in the cat's soft fur and whispered, 'I love you, Sweetie.'

After they had gone, feeling horribly sad, I gave him his final injection and stroked his head as he slipped quietly away.

CHAPTER SIXTEEN

A Cheeky Chicken, a Daft Duck and Piles of Puppies

'You're going to what?'

'Spay a duck,' Sue replied, suppressing a smile.

'How do you do that?' I said, incredulous. 'I've never heard of anyone spaying a duck. And why would you do it?'

'Because it's got egg peritonitis. You've probably come across it in chickens. The eggs keep getting stuck in the abdomen and are a prime medium for bacteria. If I spay the duck the problem's solved. And I can do it, because we've got a new machine that will allow us to anaesthetise it more effectively.'

I was fascinated. To spay a cat or dog is very straight-forward, but the problem with birds is that they are noto-riously hard to anaesthetise because they have several air sacs as well as lungs. As the anaesthetic gas is heavier than air, it gets stuck in the air sacs and then you can't wake the bird easily because it stays in the system a long time. Birds also breathe using their chest wall instead of a diaphram, so they easily tire under anaesthetic. But, as Sue explained, the new mechanical ventilator was able to deliver controlled breaths containing anaesthetic gas, which meant the bird didn't need to breathe for itself, and it helped the gas keep moving instead of settling in the air sacs.

I was back at Dacre House, the small-animal practice in Tunbridge Wells, and owner Sue was keen to keep the practice at the cutting edge of developments and to try out new procedures.

The duck in question was called Jemima and she was a real character; I could see why her owners were so fond of her that they were happy to pay for surgery. She flip-flopped around the practice on her big webbed feet, following us around like a little dog. She absolutely loved attention, quacking with delight the minute you stopped to talk to her.

Sue carried out the operation later that day, and it was a complete success. The ovaries and the uterus came out, which meant Jemima would never lay an egg again, but that didn't matter, she was a much-loved pet.

It was exciting to think that new innovations were happening all the time. Even in the few months since I'd graduated there were developments that would help save the lives of more animals.

It was mid-May and I was getting excited about my next trip. I had signed up to go to Morocco for two weeks at the beginning of June to work with a charity caring for the working animals of the world. SPANA – the Society for the Protection of Animals Abroad – run a clinic in Marrakech and a centre in Chemaia and I was going to spend a week or so in each alongside local vets treating the working horses, donkeys and mules that are part of the livelihood of many local people.

In the meantime I was working hard, dividing my weeks between three different practices. As well as working with my old friends at Dacre House, I had started as a locum a couple of days a week at Williamson's, a medium-sized practice in north Kent. And on the few spare days I had I was working for Rachel, a self-employed freelance vet who worked out of the back of her jeep visiting the homes of her clients in a rural area in East Kent.

Rachel was energetic and lively, but she was also desperate for a break. As a one-woman band her practice, built up over the previous five years, had become more successful than she'd anticipated. She was so busy that she hadn't had any time off for ages. She had called me a few weeks earlier and said she could do with some help. I was interested, so we met in a café and got to know one another over tea and cake.

'I love the job, Jo,' she told me. 'But it's hard to take a break, so if you could help me out, that would be fantastic. I'd like to spend a bit of time with my husband and children and I need to do some training workshops to keep up with the latest developments.'

I really liked the idea of visiting clients at home and driving around the lovely Kent countryside all day. So once Rachel had introduced me to a few of her regular clients, she took a couple of days off and I got going.

The reality of working on my own was harder than I had imagined. With no receptionist or nurse I had to do everything myself, beginning with fielding all the calls. Rachel had given me a list of consults for the day and her work phone. After pulling off the road to answer it a couple of times I soon learned that it was better to let it go to voicemail and then listen to the message as soon as possible. That way I could decide whether it was an emergency I needed to fit in straight away, or an appointment I could book in for later.

Following Rachel's strategy, I saw one client every hour. That allowed 30 minutes' driving time, 20 minutes with the client and 10 minutes to pack my kit into the car and grab a cup of tea or a sandwich.

On my second day I arrived to see a horse that needed vaccinating. I got out of my car and looked around, but there was no one in the stable yard, just a few chickens and a tethered horse. I watched in fascination as one of the chickens, obviously the daredevil in the flock, flapped up onto the back of the horse, climbed up to its neck and stood there, surveying the yard and no doubt enjoying the elevated view. The horse looked a little unhappy, but didn't object. It was obviously a regular arrangement, although one that was clearly favoured more by the chicken than the horse.

I was watching this little scenario – the chicken still happily atop the horse with no intention, it seemed, of coming down anytime soon – when a young man came rushing over, apologising for not being there to meet me.

'Wait a minute,' he said. 'It's Jo, isn't it?'

'Oh my goodness. Sean? I haven't seen you since …'

'Primary school,' we said in unison, laughing. Sean and I had been in the same year group at our primary school. He and his best friend Liam were always the naughty ones, disrupting class, regularly getting the dreaded blue stars that signalled trouble.

As one of the shy, good girls with my neat hairband and my prep all done, I thought Sean was very daring.

Now things had changed; I was more confident and he had clearly mellowed into a nice, laid-back man.

'You haven't changed much in the past 14 years,' he said.

'Really? Hope I don't still look 11!'

270

'No, no, I meant you look great, it's nice to see you. And you're a vet now. Guess I shouldn't be surprised, I remember you loved horses.'

'I still do. What about you? What are you up to these days?'

'Well, I've just started up my own company. It's mainly working in computer technology.'

'Something I know nothing about then! So am I here to see your horse?'

'Oh, no, it's my girlfriend's horse actually. She couldn't get here so she asked me to come and meet you.'

As we walked through the yard to the stable and I vaccinated the horse, we carried on chatting about school, old friends and our lives now. Inevitably we had lost touch with most of the people we knew as children, so it was good to look back and reminisce.

Eventually I looked at my watch. 'I'm late for my next appointment, I'd better go.'

'Good to see you, Jo,' he said. 'I knew you'd do something worthwhile.'

'Thanks, Sean, good to see you, too.'

Driving towards my next appointment – another horse vaccination – I was startled when Rachel's work phone rang. When I reached a small layby five minutes later I pulled over to check the message.

'It's Mrs Simpkins. My dog's been attacked by two huge dogs in the park. She's covered in blood and she's shaking and crying. I really need you to see her straight away.'

I called the number. 'Hello, Mrs Simpkins? It's the vet here, Jo Hardy, I'm standing in for Rachel. What's your address? I'll come straight over.'

Luckily she didn't live far away. Fifteen minutes later I pulled up outside a pretty rose-covered cottage. Mrs Simpkins must have been looking out for me, because she had the front door open while I was still unlatching the gate.

She looked distressed. 'Millie is in here. I've wrapped her in a blanket, but I didn't dare try to clean the blood off her, I thought I'd better wait for you.'

Millie was a toy poodle. Her small fluffy white head with big brown eyes peeked out of a bright orange blanket on the sofa.

'Hello, Millie, let's take a look at you.' As I carefully unwrapped the blanket I asked Mrs Simpkins what had happened.

'We were in the park going for a walk,' she said, looking down at Millie and wringing her hands. 'Suddenly these two enormous dogs pinned poor Millie down and started attacking her. They were ferocious. It was ghastly and I really thought they were going to kill her. The dogs' owner managed to get one dog off and I got the other off, though

I have no idea how, it was enormous. Millie was howling in pain and there was blood everywhere.'

As she talked I was checking Millie for injuries. She had several cuts, but I was pretty sure there were no broken bones. I cleaned her up and with the blood washed off she looked a lot less alarming.

After treating her cuts I gave her pain relief and antibiotics and told Mrs Simpkins that I would call in again the next day to see how Millie was doing. 'She'll need peace and quiet and rest, but I think she'll be fine,' I said.

Millie had a lucky escape – and so had the young Airedale terrier I was called out to see later that afternoon. A bouncy, happy dog, Rusty seemed very pleased with himself after snapping up and swallowing, in one enormous gulp, a ball of goose fat wrapped in cling film. 'I just left it on the side for a minute,' apologised the red-faced man who opened the door. 'He's not mine, I'm watching him for a friend. I'm a caterer and I was about to prepare some duck confit. Will he be OK?'

Neither the cling film nor the goose fat would do Rusty any good; I needed to make him bring it all back up as quickly as possible. I gave him an injection of apomorphine, which makes a dog throw up within minutes.

Sure enough, a few minutes later he stopped bouncing round, drooped and then started vomiting – all over the kitchen floor. We managed to get him out into the garden, which was just as well because he went on being sick intermittently for the next hour. Each time he'd feel better for a few minutes, start bouncing back, and then wilt again and throw up.

By the end of the hour absolutely everything in his stomach was out – including the goose fat and the cling film. He looked ever so sorry for himself, as if to ask what he did to deserve feeling so awful.

I helped his minder clean up the kitchen floor and then advised him to let Rusty rest a bit and to feed him normally the next day. 'There shouldn't be any after-effects,' I reassured him. 'But I guess the duck confit is off the menu.'

He smiled a wry smile. 'Mmm, I'll have to come up with something else. And watch Rusty like a hawk.'

After my encounter with Rusty I arrived home smelling gruesome, which delighted Roxy, who leaped up at me in great excitement. I must have reeked of strange dogs and vomit, clearly a heady aroma to a spaniel.

I showered and changed, grabbed a bite to eat and then Roxy and I headed off to her agility class. Mum had taken her while I was away, and we'd started going together again since I got back. I enjoyed it; we had a lot of fun and Roxy was a natural at some of the exercises. She was so good at jumping, going through tunnels and climbing that the instructor sometimes asked us to demonstrate to the class.

So far so good, but when it came to weaving, or the see-saw, Roxy still hated it. I think it must have made her feel extremely nervous, because she flatly refused to try either. The instructor lent me some weaves to set up in the garden so that we could practice at home.

I had avoided telling anyone in the class that I was a vet, but that week a new member of the class turned up – one of the nurses from Downe's, the practice where I'd been working a couple of weeks earlier. The game was up, and by the end of the class three people came up to say, 'I hear you're a vet, is there any chance you could look at my dog …?'

The following day, after making a few calls for Rachel and then nipping home for supper, I was back at Williamson's by 9pm for a night shift. It's a medium-sized, friendly practice with a good-sized hospital wing and a branch surgery a few miles away. 'We've got a little room with a bed in it just off the hospital wing, so you can sleep,' head vet Patrick had said when he first showed me around.

I'd already done three days there the previous week, but this was my first night. 'We've had a new patient in this evening,' said Roz, one of the senior vets, who was going through the patients with me before heading home. 'Oscar is a Labrador who came in after eating something toxic. He's on a drip and he seems settled in his cage, but he'll need regular checks. Rosie, one of the nurses will be in at seven in the morning. Lots of luck, hope you have a peaceful night.'

After looking in on the patients – Oscar and a couple of cats – I settled into bed, read for a while and then snoozed. I was woken a couple of hours later by a tremendous racket from the hospital room. I leaped up and rushed through to find that Oscar had pulled the drip out of his leg and somehow managed to get out of his cage. He was running round the room, slowly dripping blood from the catheter site, waking the cats and no doubt wondering how to get home.

'Oh Oscar,' I said. 'What have you done?'

It took me an hour to get hold of him, put in another drip – which he made it clear he most definitely did not want by wriggling like crazy – get him back into his cage and settled, and then clean up the bloody paw-prints he'd left all over the place. By that time it was after 2am and my shoulder, still sore from the wrench Tammy had given it, was aching. Rubbing it, I crawled back into bed, hoping to get a few more hours' sleep.

As a result of the night's antics I was a little bleary-eyed the next morning when I arrived at the Williamson's branch surgery, where I was doing the first session. It was a small prefab, with just two rooms: one for the reception area and a consulting room.

First in that morning was a very grumpy man with a collie, in for a kennel cough vaccination.

'Where's Jason, the regular vet?' he said.

'He's on holiday, I'm standing in,' I told him.

'Well, you won't be able to do this because my dog likes a man to give him the vaccine. He isn't keen on women.'

'I'm sure I'll be fine,' I said firmly, feeling a little taken aback. But the grumpy owner was right – the collie took one look at me with the syringe in my hand and hurled itself around the small room like a creature demented, as the owner struggled to get it under control. We did manage in the end, but it took quite some time for me to get near enough to administer the squirt of vaccine up the nose, and when I did the dog sneezed, violently, right in my face.

'Thanks,' I muttered under my breath.

That afternoon I was back at the Williamson's main surgery, doing the 4pm till 7pm session. It was actually pretty quiet. I had a couple of minor cases until, just after 6pm, a couple, Jed and Hannah, arrived with their young springer spaniel, which was in the middle of giving birth. She'd had four puppies, which they brought with them wrapped in towels in a cardboard box, but she hadn't passed another for a couple of hours and they were worried.

'We're sure there's more,' said Jed. 'The way she's acting, pacing around and stressed, we think she's waiting for another.'

'We can scan her and try to see what's there,' I said. I called Roz, who was in the next room. Together we took the springer, Sasha, in for a scan.

'There's definitely another puppy there,' Roz said. She was right. I could see it on the scan, and when I examined Sasha I could feel the sack around the puppy with the end of my rubber-gloved finger.

'It's just going to be a question of waiting at this stage,' Roz said. 'Jo, will you stay with them? I'll be nearby if you need me.'

I sat with Jed and Hannah, drinking cups of tea and watching Sasha, who alternately slumped, paced restlessly or sniffed at her four puppies, which were mewling in their box. Every 30 minutes I gave her an injection of oxytocin, which helps with contractions.

An hour later, Roz popped her head in. 'Any progress?'

'No,' we all chorused.

'OK, well, let's give her one more injection and wait another 20 minutes and then we'll have to do a caesarean. I'll operate and, Jo, the nurses have gone home so I'll need your help.'

Jed and Hannah were a little alarmed by the prospect of an operation. 'It's very straightforward,' I told them. 'And if she carries on trying to give birth for too long she'll be in distress and the remaining puppy will be in danger. She will still be able to feed the puppies, but because of the incision she might be a bit sore. If she seems to be uncomfortable you can get artificial puppy milk; it's just going to be a lot of work for you, I'm afraid.'

'That's OK,' said Hannah. 'It's her first litter, you know. We came over from New Zealand to live in the UK for three years – we're both doing postgrad research work – and we just had to have a dog. We found Sasha through a rescue charity. She was just a few months old. We'll take her home with us when we go back.'

'And the puppies?' I asked. 'Will you sell them?'

'Sell or give, yes,' Hannah said. 'But we might keep one, for Sasha, and because, well, who can resist a puppy?'

A cup of tea later and there was still no change, so we left Jed and Hannah with the puppies to look after and keep warm and took Sasha through to the operating suite.

Once she was anaesthetised Roz made an incision down her belly and within seconds she had lifted out a puppy – a fairly large one, too. I took it and wrapped it in a warm towel, rubbing it firmly on the back to dry it off and stimulate breathing.

'There's more,' she said. 'In fact … there are two more.' And out came two more bruisers.

'Wow, three large puppies. No wonder Sasha was tired,' I said.

When Sasha was stitched up and resting, we took the puppies through to Jed and Hannah.

'She had seven?' Jed said, incredulous. 'And we might need to feed all of them? It's goodbye sleep, I guess.' He and Hannah didn't know whether to laugh or cry – in fact, they did both.

It was almost 10 by the time we'd finished and Sasha was awake. We gave her back her puppies, which she started to nuzzle, and told Jed and Hannah we'd keep her in for the next 24 hours to monitor them. All being well, she would go home the next day with plenty of dried puppy milk in case she was too sore to feed.

'I've had an amazing day,' I told Mum as I wolfed down a plate of shepherd's pie. 'I was wondering – what would you think about getting another springer puppy? I've seen some today that are just sooo sweet, and I'm sure Roxy would love it.'

'Jo, are you mad?' Mum said. 'Roxy most definitely would not want to share her humans with an upstart newcomer! Like a lot of rescues she's a bit insecure. I find it hard enough resisting bringing home some of the dogs I collect from the pound. I couldn't have another dog unless it was a rescue.'

I sighed. She was right, of course. But that night, as I drifted into an exhausted sleep, I couldn't help thinking that, against all logic, a puppy just melts your heart.

CHAPTER SEVENTEEN

Morocco

Through the scrum of people milling through Marrakech airport I spotted a small, round, elderly man with silver hair holding up a sign with my name on it.

I approached him. '*Bonjour, je m'apelle* Jo. *Parlez-vous anglais?*' He shook his head and carried on smiling.

I wasn't sure how far my schoolgirl French was going to get me. '*Je voudrais un SIM,*' I said, pointing to my phone. Nothing. I started taking my phone apart to show him the SIM card.

'Ah, OK,' he nodded, and he led me towards a shop where, luckily, the assistant spoke English, had the right SIM and installed it for me.

We left the airport and the old man, who told me, with much gesticulating, that his name was Boujema, took me to a lorry that stank of horses. I had to be in the right place.

The chaotic traffic we drove through reminded me of Uganda, but everything else was very different. Marrakech is a major city, with grand hotels, stunning palaces, mosques and public gardens, as well as a maze of poorer quarters.

I stared out of the window, fascinated by glimpses of street markets, ornately carved doors and women in brightly coloured robes. Eventually we left the city behind and reached the SPANA clinic, where I would be working, on the outskirts of town.

Situated inside a walled compound, it was like a little oasis away from the busy city. We drove in through the gates to a central courtyard where several peacocks and peahens strutted about on a grassy area. Boujema, who was the centre's driver, helped me unload my suitcase and pointed me in the direction of the accommodation.

The building was bigger and grander than I had imagined it would be, although I knew that SPANA, a British charity dedicated to helping the working animals of the world, aims to put the highest-standard facilities in parts of the world where the animals need help. They don't aim to make the best of a bad situation – they aim to make the situation far better. In Morocco they have five centres, each run by Moroccan vets. These vets also have their own private practices, so when English vets come out to help it really makes a difference.

I was shown around by Samir, who introduced himself as a horse technician who assisted the vets.

I was impressed by the facilities. There were 26 hospital boxes, most of which were full, plus two examination areas with stocks for the horses. There was even a padded knock-down box for performing surgeries and a small paddock.

I stayed in one of several bedrooms next to the stables. My room was small, just big enough for the single bed and a suitcase. It opened onto a courtyard area and just across the courtyard was a kitchen and bathroom.

In the room next to mine was another vet, Chloe, who had arrived earlier that day. She had graduated a few years earlier and had come out to Morocco in a break between jobs. After a bit of time in mixed practice she had special-ised as an equine vet.

We liked one another straight away. Chloe was a sporty country girl. She had cycled from London to Paris and had worked with another charity, at a horse and donkey trust in Gambia. I noted it for future reference, as it sounded like somewhere I would love to go.

The clinic was within walking distance of the shops and cafés, so that evening Chloe and I walked to a little restau-rant for dinner. The food was delicious, and very cheap.

I was tired and ready for a good night's sleep, but I hadn't counted on the peacocks. They shrieked, all night long. I thought I loved peacocks, but by morning I'd decided I definitely didn't. They might be pretty, but they were noisier than cockerels, and their din was accompanied by the sporadic whinnying and braying of the donkeys and horses in the boxes.

By morning I was bleary-eyed and cursing peacocks. Chloe and I met in the kitchen for a breakfast of orange juice and pastries and she looked as tired as I felt.

'Apparently peacocks are incredibly popular in Morocco,' she said. 'I can't think why.'

Tired or not, we needed to start work. By 8.30am a second vet technician, Omar, was ready to take us with him on his morning round and to introduce us to our patients. The horses had already been fed, watered and mucked out. As we went from horse box to horse box, with Omar checking charts, temperatures and medications, he explained to us that as vet technicians he and Samir, who did the later shift, could do intravenous injections, put horses on drips, put in nasogastric tubes for horses with colic and wash and dress wounds. I was impressed. He seemed knowledgeable and capable, and with him and Samir to keep things running the vet only needed to come out to the clinic for a few hours a day to do new consultations and to check on inpatients.

After rounds we spent the next couple of hours washing wounds and bandaging legs, bringing each horse out to the stocks to be treated. The majority of the inpatients had injuries from the carts they pulled, from their harnesses or from accidents. Some of the wounds we treated were appalling. One horse had lost a large area of skin from his rump. It was far too big an area to cover with any kind of bandage so, Omar explained, we simply had to clean it every day and let it heal. Many of the injuries were so severe that in England the animal would have been put to sleep, but in Morocco euthanasia was frowned upon, both for religious reasons and because each animal was vital to the livelihood of a family.

By late morning there would be a long queue of people waiting to see the vet. Their animals were tethered to a long chain strung between two poles inside the gates. Most of the owners would bring their horses and donkeys there early, go away for a few hours and come back when the vet arrived.

The vet, Mohamed, one of two who worked at the clinic, arrived and thanked us warmly for coming, before informing us he would be doing small animal consults on-site, leaving us to take charge of equine things with Omar. As each horse, donkey or mule was led across the yard, Chloe and I examined it and tried to treat it after numerous questions to Omar about what medications he had available. We dealt with colic cases, lameness – a lot of them had shoes made of rubber from old tyres – and bad teeth. Many of them had never had their teeth rasped and so they had become uneven and sharp. Chloe was an expert in equine dentistry, so she dealt with most of those cases.

After the consults Mohamed checked that we were happy with our morning's work and then left, so Chloe and I caught a taxi into the city to have lunch. In the heat of the day a cheap taxi was preferable to a long, hot walk.

Lunch gave us a welcome break. The afternoon was quieter than the morning, but there were still more horses and more procedures, operations and routine checks. The clinic was incredibly busy, and the majority of the horse boxes were occupied most of the time, although we did manage to go into the city and explore some of the fascinating souks, the street markets filled with spices and delicious foods, and the little alleyways and paths of the old city.

One of our first serious cases was a little bay stallion with a pretty pony face. We called him Little Bay, as horses don't have names in Morocco. He came into the clinic in a bad way; his gums were pale, his temperature was through the roof, he was dehydrated and he had a horrendous cough, although we weren't sure whether this was related to his other symptoms or whether two different things were going on. I took some blood and stained it up to look at it under the microscope. The red blood cells were crawling with babesia, a protozoal parasite transmitted by ticks. It was the same illness I had seen in the dogs in South Africa.

Little Bay's owner, who used the horse to pull his cart of wares, was very concerned. He stood watching anxiously as we swung into action to treat his animal. We started with antibiotics that were strong enough to treat both the babesia and the cough, as well as some pain relief, but then Little Bay suddenly flung himself on the floor, panicking us all. We gave him a sedative and more pain relief and inserted a catheter and a drip to give him intravenous fluids because he was so dehydrated.

He had arrived looking terrible – I honestly thought he was dying – but an hour later he was bright, comfortable, happy and looking for attention, as if to say, 'I'm fine, sorry I frightened you!' It was a scary colic reaction, but Mohamed assured us he sometimes saw that with the antibiotic we had given because it causes spasms in the gut wall.

Little Bay wasn't out of the woods yet, though, and over the next few days he alternated between looking very ill and much brighter. His owner came in every day with extra hay for him, staying to talk to him and stroke him. Many of the owners were devoted to their animals – their horse or donkey was part of the family, and their value was clearly much more than just financial.

At the end of our first week Chloe and I took a Sunday off to hike up the Atlas Mountains.

We took a tourist bus there, thinking it would be a gentle hike, but in fact it turned out to be a climb up a sheer mountain, with dozens of other tourists on the same route, all climbing on top of each other.

There were a couple of other European people in our group who seemed quite confident, but they hit difficulties halfway up and decided they couldn't go on. Chloe and I pressed on, though, and got almost to the top. There was a waterfall there, in seven different parts, and a little shop. And of course the view was stunning. Our guide told us that if we could just get up to the next level there was a much better way down, but to do it we had to pay the shop-keeper to let us use his ladder to get up a sheer rock face. We made it, and the guide was right. The view was even more spectacular and we came down on a different, paral-lel path that was easier.

For our second week Chloe and I transferred to one of SPANA's other centres, in Chemaia. This was a small town to the west of Marrakech, and we travelled there in a grand taxi (these were for longer trips, while the petit taxis were for local journeys). The taxi was an ancient yellow Mercedes and the driver waited until it was full before he would go. That meant four other people in addition to him, Chloe and me – seven of us plus luggage in all. One very cramped hour later we were there.

The SPANA centre at Chemaia was half the size of the one in Marrakech, but just as nice. There were 12 hospitalisation stables and a stock for procedures. A very charismatic technician called Driss showed us around and introduced us to the two highly experienced vets, Youness and Kamal. All three were so welcoming that they made us feel part of the team the moment we arrived.

The order of the day was very similar to how it had been in Marrakech, but if anything we were even busier. By the time we'd done the morning medications and checked all the critical patients, washed wounds, rebandaged and made sure that all the horses got some grass from the patch at the front, it was lunchtime. The shops were too far away, so Driss would make us egg sandwiches and tea. He would chat to people who came in with their horses and carts to drink at the water trough placed at the front gate, and distribute fluorescent headcollars, bridles and plates to go on the back of the cart so that they would be more visible to cars in poor light. This project is unique to Chemaia and incredibly popular. The staff there asked SPANA to fund it and they agreed. Now most horses and carts are kitted out in hi-vis!

At about 2pm the consults would start. We would work alongside either Kamal or Youness, as legally a British vet isn't allowed to make the decisions in Morocco unless a Moroccan vet is also on-site. Kamal was only there when needed, but Youness came for a few hours a day. Driss told him, 'We have English vets now, you go.' He was saying, don't worry, they are capable – you can have a rest. If anything needed to change, we would ring the Moroccan vets for them to come back and assess and make the decision officially. After that, Chloe and I were left in charge quite a lot of the time, outside the regular consulting times.

After consults, any major procedures and stitch-ups were done and the day would finish some time between 4.30 and 6.30pm. After that, Chloe and I would usually head down to a local restaurant for a salad and tagine, then relax for a couple of hours before night-time checks and meds at about 10pm. We'd fall asleep quickly, exhausted and exhilarated from the day.

We treated dozens of cases, but among those that stayed with me long afterwards was the heavily pregnant little donkey with colic who we named Julia. On examination we realised that her uterus had become twisted. In England she would have been referred to an animal hospital for specialist surgery or put to sleep, but I realised Youness and Kamal were clipping her flank for surgery. My first thoughts were, They have to be kidding! How on earth are they going to do a caesarean and correct the torsion as a standing surgery? But while I administered the sedative, they cracked on bravely with it.

This was what in England we call superhero surgery – something extraordinary that was rare and risky. But they pulled it off. Youness delivered the foal – sadly dead, as the twist had cut off his blood supply – and then he and Kamal between them located the twist in her uterus, untwisted it and stitched her back up. Julia, heavily sedated, stood stoically and bravely throughout while her owner, a tall, elderly man, stayed throughout, sitting on a chair in front of her with her head on his lap, stroking her nose.

Unsurprisingly she got bad peritonitis (inflammation of the abdomen) afterwards, but with decent pain relief, a shed-load of antibiotics and intravenous fluids she pulled through. As she got better we realised she was quite a character – bossy and quite stubborn, but a real fighter too. Throughout her convalescence her owner, who doted on her, brought her fresh greenery every day.

Another special case was Maggie, a donkey who came in with colic. Her heart rate (normally under 44 for a donkey) was 100. She was massively dehydrated and when we drew out some of her abdominal fluid, instead of a clearish liquid, it was dark brown. Chloe and I would have expected to put her to sleep, but in Morocco, unless the animal looks dead, it can't be put to sleep, as the vets would be considered animal killers and would lose respect from the public. So instead we put her on lots of IV fluids, passed a stomach tube every few hours to check she wasn't refluxing, then added more fluids and put her on a high dose of pain relief. Surprisingly, the next morning she was a little better. She was still quiet and not eating, but her heart rate was now in the 60s. Over the week she fluctuated, but she did slowly improve and even started to pick at grass when turned out with other donkeys. She was a very sociable animal and always looked brighter when she was around others, so we'd make sure that she got a bit of time with the other donkeys every day.

My favourite of all we called Sophie. She was a tiny donkey who collapsed in the street while pulling her cart, presumably from exhaustion. It then ran over her, causing massive trauma to her face and knees. Chloe and I spent an afternoon suturing her face back together. She had lost a lot of skin and some of the bone underneath was damaged, so it was a long procedure, but we managed it and afterwards she looked a bit more respectable, if a little battered. The main complication, though, was that she had damaged the nerve to the left eyelid, as well as the muscles above her left eye, so she couldn't blink or close that eye. However, most animals have a third eyelid; a thin pinky-coloured membranous skin on the inside of the eyelid, and luckily Sophie still had control of this, although her new way of blinking made her look like a lizard. Her outer eyelids would remain still, while the pink membrane underneath would slide down over her eye.

We pampered and fussed over her, cleaning her wounds every day, squirting water into her eyes to keep them lubricated, keeping up her antibiotics and pain relief and giving her lots of her favourite treat – watermelon rind. The horses and donkeys in Morocco loved this, but when we bought them apples and carrots as treats, they didn't know what to do with them.

It was extraordinary what the horses and donkeys in Morocco endured, but despite their resilience, every now and then there was a case so severe that not even the gallant vets and technicians could do anything to help. While I was at Chemaia, a transit van pulled up with a horse in the back. The poor creature had a swinging leg fracture – a leg broken so badly that it was impossible to treat. I had to turn away and take a deep breath to compose myself when I saw it. We had no idea how they'd got the horse into the van, and we had to get it out again, which was shocking in itself, as the horse had to jump down onto the ground. Finally we managed to get it out and hold it still while we placed a mattress next to it. It fell over on the mattress as we put it to sleep. I was so grateful that we were able to end its pain.

That happened on a Friday, which is the holy day in Morocco, which made it even harder for the owner. Driss spent a lot of time consoling him.

Chloe and I were touched by what a caring culture we found in Morocco, with everyone giving what they could to the less fortunate. We decided to become part of that, so we bought bread every day to give to those who needed it.

At the end of our week Chloe went to join her boyfriend for a week of surfing on the coast, and I went back to Marrakech for five more days. This time I met the second SPANA vet, Boubka, who had been away at a conference when we had first been there at the start of our trip.

Boubka turned out to be fantastic to work with and very trusting of my ability. The first day we worked together, he showed me a donkey that had suffered a horrific injury. He was the smallest adult donkey I had ever seen, so I had to call him Tiny. The donkey's back leg had been de-gloved; in other words the skin had been stripped right off the leg after an injury at the top of the leg. I couldn't bear to think how it had happened, or how much it must hurt.

Boubka anaesthetised him in the knock-down box, told me I was going to reconstruct his leg and then left me to it. The only companion I had was one of the cleaners, a tall middle-aged man who didn't speak much English and who stood silently to one side, ready to run for help if I needed it.

It took the whole afternoon. I couldn't just flap the skin back up over the wound and stitch along the edge, as there would have been a lot of open space underneath where the skin wouldn't be attached to the muscle. To make sure it adhered down to the muscle, I put a stitch through the skin and muscle at regular intervals, then back through the skin and then tied it through a button. It is an old-school technique in England, but it works.

At the end I stood back, happy with my work. When Tiny came round, we moved him into a horse box and nursed him with great care. I got to know him well over my last few days; he was kind-natured, always quick to say hello and wanting to please. He always put his ears forwards in greeting and seemed happy and he never put up a fuss when I was cleaning his wound.

Tiny made it back to his delighted owner, and while I was sorry to see him go, I was so happy that he was recovering.

The next case Boubka gave me was a very naughty mule foal who was still growing into his ears. In the stable he was fine, although he always tried to pick your pockets for treats, but outside and in the stocks all he wanted to do was jump around. He didn't know the meaning of still. The foal had an umbilical hernia, which needed to be surgically corrected by opening him up, pushing the hernia back into his abdomen and closing the hole in the muscle wall that it was coming through. I had never performed this surgery in practice, although I had helped to do it once as a student, but Boubka decided that was good enough. I knew how to do it and I had plenty of surgical experience from the UK on small animals so, again, he knocked out the foal for me and pretty much left me to it. There was no monitor on the anaesthetic, which was set up as a continuous drip into his neck, so they told me to 'just shout if the animal moves, runs out of drip or starts waking up'. The technicians were nearby and once again the cleaner stayed with me to act as my runner. This time I had to get him to go and find the vet when it looked as though the drip was going to run out before I'd completed the surgery. Boubka came, set up a new drip and went back to looking after the new cases coming in. I was really pleased that he trusted me and I was happy with the final result, although I don't think the foal was quite so impressed after that ordeal! Despite that, he made a full recovery and when last I saw him he was leaping around in the paddock.

I learned so much during my time in Morocco, and while there my confidence grew thanks to Boubka, the Chemaia vets and all the kind and competent technicians. They were all extraordinary people, giving so much time and effort to help others by treating their working horses, mules and donkeys who are so important to them. They constantly pushed the boundaries of their own expertise to save the lives of these animals. I was sorry to say goodbye.

CHAPTER EIGHTEEN

Wedding Plans and Lucy's Surprise

It was absolutely perfect. I knew the minute I saw it that this was the place where Jacques and I should hold our wedding reception.

I was standing in a beautiful rustic converted barn with Abi and my parents. The ceilings were high, there was a balcony overlooking the main hall and it would easily fit 100 people eating, dancing and celebrating.

Jacques and I had set a date for our wedding and at last it was beginning to feel real. We'd chosen early autumn the following year and although that was not for another 16 months, as everyone kept telling me and I was beginning to realise, that was not really so far ahead with so much to do and plan.

I knew that Jacques would have liked an African bush wedding, but he knew that I wanted to marry among my friends and family in England, so in the end we had agreed to marry in England and have a second celebration, a reception, later on in South Africa. Some of his family and friends would fly over for the English ceremony, and some of mine would fly to South Africa for the reception there.

Before I went to Morocco I had started looking around for a church to marry in and a venue for the reception. The church we settled on was in Wadhurst, a beautiful little village not far from us. It would be decorated for the harvest festival, in yellows and oranges, and I planned to add more flowers in purples and pinks to make it, I hope, a riot of beautiful sunset colours.

We wanted our wedding to be fun, country-style, and a big party for everyone to enjoy – nothing too formal or pretentious. The barn I was looking at with Abi and my parents seemed perfect; it was only a few miles from the church and their chef said he would be happy to cook South African food. I hope we'll have *potjie*, which is a beef casserole, in cauldrons on each table so that people can serve each other.

At every step I was excitedly Skyping Jacques, who said all the right things, although we both knew that he was happy for me to make most of the decisions. He trusted me, and there were only a few aspects of the arrangements that he felt strongly about. His main job was planning a honeymoon for us – and keeping it a surprise, so that I wouldn't know where we were going until we set off. I promised I would leave it to him and not interfere – much! – but I did rule out a bush safari, just in case that was what he was thinking of. I hoped we would go somewhere that neither of us had ever been before.

My biggest challenge was finding the right dress. Mum and I had started going to bridal shops and looking through the racks, and although I tried on lots of dresses, none were right. I didn't want a meringue; I wanted flowing, elegant and original. The weekend before I flew to Morocco, we went to a sale of sample bridal dresses in a tiny bridal boutique where everyone was rushing to grab the dresses from the rail. I really didn't expect to find anything – but then I saw it: an absolutely lovely dress. I tried it on, and Mum burst into tears. We'd found the one!

It was glamorous and gorgeous with a slight boho look to it as well. With flowers in my hair it would look perfect. The only snag was that it was far too big. But I knew some-one at the stables where my horses were who was brilliant at alterations.

With the dress safely tucked away at home – and Dad breathing a sigh of relief because we'd got it in a sale – I knew everything else would fall into place. Of course, we still had to sort out the small matter of which country we would live in once we were married, but we still had time to decide that. And I would be seeing Jacques soon – he and his parents were coming over in early July for a holiday. Although my parents and Jacques's had exchanged friendly emails, they hadn't yet met, so we had planned a week in Cornwall for both families together, so that they could get to know each other. I was pretty sure they would all get on, but that didn't stop me feeling nervous as the holiday drew nearer.

I had two very full weeks of work booked in before Jacques and his parents arrived, but first I was looking forward to a long-overdue catch-up with Lucy.

We had dinner one Saturday evening, halfway between her house and mine, and the moment she walked in I could see that something was up. She looked great, and she couldn't stop smiling.

'What's up?' I asked, trying not to sound too suspicious.

'What do you mean?' she said, trying to look innocent.

'You look different. Happy. Very happy.'

'I'm always happy.' Still innocent.

'Not this happy. You're … glowing.'

'OK, well, I've just finished my internship and been confirmed in a permanent job. So yes, I'm very happy!'

'Oh Lucy, that's wonderful, I'm so glad for you. We have to drink a toast.'

'And there's more … I've met someone.'

'You what? Oh wow. I knew something was up. I want every single tiny little detail. Starting with his name.'

'It's Ant, and he's lovely. We met when one of the farmers set me up on a blind date.'

I was hooked. I couldn't wait to hear the whole story, and Lucy obliged, telling me how she had been visiting one of her regular farms, pregnancy scanning the cows, when the farmer asked whether she had a boyfriend. 'A few minutes later he said he might have a friend he could set me up with.'

Lucy had blushed scarlet and stuttered that she didn't need to be set up, but the farmer had insisted and had organised for Lucy and the mystery man to come over for supper.

On the way there Lucy stopped to take a call in a gateway and managed to reverse into the end of the gate so that the latch sheared the side of her car's rear bumper. Needless to say, by the time she got to the farmer's house she was feeling a bit flustered.

Ant, the farmer's friend, seemed very nice, and at the end of the evening he took her number. Lucy carried on with the story.

'As I left the farmer came out to check his cows and spotted my car, to great hilarity. He told most of the other farmers in the area about the vet who had crashed her car on the way to his house for a double date with his friend.'

Despite all the mishaps Lucy agreed to a date with Ant – but had to cancel twice, after which they eventually managed a coffee and a walk with the dog.

'And …?' I was all ears.

'After the third date, which was mercifully incident-free, I linked my hand in his as we walked back to the car after having an epic Chinese meal. We shared a quick kiss and my stomach did all the right sort of flipping.'

'What a great story. What does he look like?'

'Oh, medium build, strawberry blond – OK, ginger, but that's cool now, right? Muscly and with a lovely smile.'

'I can't wait to meet him.'

'You will. How are the wedding plans?'

'Coming along, I have a dress …'

'You have to show me. Have you decided about brides-maids' dresses? Because I'm not doing anything frilly.'

'You know I wouldn't make you wear frills. Just a few bows …'

She looked so horrified I wished I could capture the moment.

'Only joking. Elegant and simple, and I thought dark purple. Is that all right?'

'Phew. That sounds good. I can start looking forward to it now.'

It was a lovely evening. I was so happy to hear about Lucy's new man, and her job. She was becoming a female James Herriot, living in a farm bubble, and it couldn't have suited her more. She always had a way with cows.

The following Monday morning I was back at Dacre House with Sue and Bradley, and now my old housemate Andrew, too. He had settled in well and although he still said he wasn't sure what he wanted to do in the long term, they liked having him there and he fitted in.

My first patient that day was a hamster named Eric. He had been found by his nine-year-old owner dangling upside down in his cage from one of the bars, affixed by a strip of bedding that had got itself wrapped around his leg. The family had cut him down but they couldn't get the strip of bedding off and it was strangulating the leg.

Watched by an anxious small girl and her mother, I managed, with a lot of difficulty, to get the strip off his leg. By this time the leg had become engorged with blood – it was a really dark red colour and there was a real possibility that he could lose it. It had been starved of blood for some time and there was a danger that his circulation wouldn't function properly again. Once I'd taken off the piece of bedding and given poor Eric pain relief, I asked the owners to bring him back a couple of days later. They phoned the next day to say he seemed in pain, but he did recover – he kept his leg, and his owners changed the type of bedding they used.

The theme that afternoon, though, was puppies. In came a whole box full of brand-new beagle puppies – five very sweet, wriggly little things. Along with their mother, they needed a post-birth examination.

I checked the puppies first, looking for cleft palates and heart murmurs. Cleft palates can be fixed and heart murmurs in new puppies often disappear within a few weeks, but these puppies had neither. I checked that their bottoms were not bunged up with meconium, the first stool they produce, and finally I checked their lungs to make sure they were nice and full of air. Puppies' lungs have no air in them at birth, so they need to fill up and begin to function normally as soon as possible after they have been born.

Having checked the puppies I turned to their mother, a lovely young beagle, clearly delighted with her first litter. I made sure that she had plenty of milk for them and no sign of inflamed mammary glands and looked to see that she had not torn during the birth. Everything was as it should be, so I sent them all home with their very pleased owner.

A couple of hours later another puppy arrived, brought in by her worried owner Annie. This time it was a tiny

Boston terrier and she was in a bad way. Just five weeks old, she was very sick and barely able to lift her head. She needed to be hospitalised while we worked out the problem. We had to put her on a drip to get some glucose and fluids into her, but she was too small, so we injected glucose solution under her skin instead. In fact, she was so tiny that she fitted into the palm of a hand – she probably weighed no more than a few ounces. Her name was Dixie and she appeared to be suffering, but it was difficult to say what the cause was. It looked as if it could be pneumonia, as her breathing seemed a bit laboured, but the main worry was that she had gone downhill pretty quickly according to her owner.

Annie left her with us and I promised to update her regularly. For the next few hours we nursed her and kept her warm. I gave her some antibiotics, in case it was an infection causing her to fade so quickly. The nurses took to carrying her around inside their tops – and she seemed to be responding to something we were doing. But I was worried, so I talked to Bradley, who was covering that night.

His wife and his small son had just been in to say hello and to bring him some food. He was about to eat when he saw how worried I looked. He asked me about what breed she was and what signs she had been showing, so I told him that she just seemed to be fading and the owner had noticed her being a bit slower than the rest. He pushed his meal to one side and quickly came to look at Dixie.

'I'm afraid we may lose her tonight,' I said. 'Is there anything else we can do?'

Bradley felt her skull.

'As I suspected, there's an open fontanelle. Feel this gap in her skull,' he said. 'Small-headed and domed-headed breeds like chihuahuas, Boston terriers, Yorkies and Pekingese, for example, are prone to fluid on the brain – hydrocephalus – and this may well be her problem. It causes the puppy to develop slowly and to be almost dumb, if the puppy survives at all, that is. Carry on giving her glucose. I know you started it because she's a puppy and needs it because she's weak, but it actually draws the fluid out of the brain so it works on two levels, and then just keep her warm on a heat pad. She needs pretty intensive nursing. I'll watch her tonight and we'll see how she is in the morning.'

Dixie may have been tiny, but she was a fighter. She made it through the night and in a couple of days she was well enough to go home. A few weeks later Bradley told me that Dixie had been back, with her brothers and sisters, for her routine vaccinations. She had been well, growing fast and full of mischief.

'We've found homes for them all,' Annie had told Bradley. 'All except Dixie. She's special, so we've decided to keep her.'

On a Monday evening in early July I made my way into London to meet Jacques's parents, Elna and Johan, for dinner. They had arrived from South Africa that morning and Jacques was coming a few days later.

After giving me a warm hello hug, Elna got straight to the point.

'My son cannot live here,' she said. 'London is just so … frightening. Everyone is looking at their phones as they walk along, and as for the tube system, I don't understand it at all.'

It didn't help that the weather was grey and gloomy. Their first trip to England and they were plainly not enjoying it. I did my best to reassure them.

'London is a bit overwhelming, I know. But don't just judge England by London – there's so much more to see and you'll love it. And if we do live here Jacques and I won't be in London, I promise.'

Elna looked relieved, while Johan nodded. We had a nice meal and they talked about the coach trip they had planned to places all over the UK during the next couple of weeks, before we all got together in Cornwall. I left them that night hoping that their first impression of

England would be swept aside once they saw some of its beauty.

While his parents travelled, Jacques flew over and came with me to look at the wedding venue and to meet the caterer, after which we drove down to Cornwall.

My family and Jacques's family were each staying in separate holiday homes, but we'd be meeting up each day to spend time together. It was a good arrangement, not too much for anyone, and with lots of time to get to know each other. One evening both sets of parents went out to dinner together while Ross, Jacques and I stayed at home with a takeaway and a film.

'How do you think it's going?' I said, every five minutes.

'Fine – I hope,' Jacques replied each time.

When they all came back at around 11pm they walked in stony-faced and said, 'That's it, the wedding's off.' We stared at them, horrified, until they all started laughing. They'd had a great time and were playing a joke on us. I had thought that Dad and Elna would get on well because they're both extroverts and that my Mum and Johan would click as they are both quieter, but actually Elna is just a chattier version of Mum, so they got on really well, swapping phone numbers and pictures of their dogs.

It was a lovely week. We ate lots of fish and chips and pasties and, when the weather was good, we went to the beach. It was Roxy's first trip to Cornwall; she had never seen the sea before. We had assumed that all springer spaniels loved water – Tosca and our previous dog, Bluff, certainly had – but Roxy ran up to it, then grabbed a mouthful of seaweed, shook it around and spat it out before running back to my parents. She tried a second time and a big wave came and sent her racing for cover again.

In the end Dad waded out knee-deep into the sea and coaxed her into the water. She went in, but she didn't know how to swim and thrashed around so Mum and Dad had to teach her how. Once she got the hang of it you couldn't get her out of the water. She was a typical springer after all.

One evening we took Jacques and his parents to Bedruthan Steps to watch the sunset. It is between Padstow and Newquay, in a National Trust conservation area, and when you stand on the top of the cliff, the sun sets directly in front of you. It's stunning.

I've taken Jacques there before; he always stands right on the edge of the cliff to take photos and his dad did exactly the same thing. The rest of us watched in horror, yelping, 'Don't go so close,' while they looked puzzled and said, 'What do you mean?'

'You're terrifying us,' I yelled, followed by Elna yelling, 'Please come away from there. You're both too close.'

'Now you know where I get it from,' Jacques replied, with his schoolboy grin, and he turned back to photographing the birds and the sunset without stepping even an inch away from the cliff edge.

Towards the end of the week Mum got a message to say that a dog she had transported had gone missing. Mum regularly works as a volunteer for charities that rescue dogs. She's part of a network of drivers who take the dogs to foster carers or new homes all over the country. Mum explained that Milo was a springer spaniel that she had transported to a foster carer a couple of weeks earlier. He was very young and scared of absolutely everything, so she hoped he was going to find a loving home where he would regain his confidence. The foster carer he went to had said that he needed rehabilitation training, but only days later he was rehomed. As soon as his new owners opened the car door, though, Milo had made a run for it. They found him, but he did it again and this time he was gone for days. As the search for him continued, a dog was spotted, scared and running, near a busy road. The searchers sent a picture of it to Mum to ask her to confirm that it was Milo. It was, and she was very worried about him.

A couple of days later we heard that they had managed to track him down and found him living wild, feeding himself on a deer carcass. It took them a while to catch him, staking out the deer carcass at night, but as soon as he was caught he was sent for the rehabilitation training he needed. He would be living with several other dogs who would show him what he needed to do, while at the same time he would be trained to go for walks off the lead and answer to recall.

Hearing that Milo was safe was a happy note at the end of our holiday. With promises to stay in touch, Jacques's parents headed for their flight home, Jacques and I headed back to Kent to meet a wedding photographer and my parents and Ross stayed on in Cornwall for a few more days.

Jacques flew back to South Africa a few days later. This time we would only be apart for a matter of weeks, as I was going to be flying out for his birthday the following month, so I managed not to flood Heathrow with my tears as I saw him off. Another year – and a bit – and we would be together, always. I couldn't wait.

By early July I had been a qualified vet for a whole year. And what an incredible year it had been, with all my travels abroad and the variety of practices I had worked in. I felt very lucky. It had been exciting, eye-opening and a wonderful start to my life as a vet.

Back at Dacre House the following week I celebrated my first year as a qualified vet by asking Bradley to sign off my records. I had carefully recorded, every day, the hundreds of cases I'd seen over the year in my Professional Development Record (PDR), which was an online record monitored by the veterinary governing body, the Royal College of Veterinary Surgeons. They had judged it good enough for me to be signed off on my first year and declared competent as a year-one vet. They had sent a certificate saying so, which a senior staffer had to sign.

I took the certificate to Bradley, who had agreed to mentor me at the start of the year. He'd just finished a night shift and after three overnight emergencies and two hours' sleep, he looked pretty tired.

'You've been competent for ages, Jo,' he said. 'You're a good vet, and I'm happy to sign you off. Now I need to get some rest.'

It will never be an easy life, being a vet.

But as long as I'm making a difference to people's lives by helping their animals, it's a good one.

Acknowledgements

I'd like to take this opportunity to mention and thank the many people who got me through this hugely tough first year of being a qualified vet. I want to especially thank my friends and family, and my wonderful other half, and soon-to-be husband, Jacques, for encouraging me through some incredibly arduous times and supporting me when I told them I wanted to go and work in remote and often dangerous areas of the world. I love you all.

I'd also like to thank the charities that supported me while I was abroad, either with inner-country assistance and housing, or with supplies and finances that I needed for the trips: World in Need, SPANA, SPCA, the Worldwide Veterinary Services, the British Goat Society, the Veterinary Christian Fellowship, the British Veterinary Association and WAHL – you are all amazing people with such generous hearts.

Also, I can't thank Kate Latham and the HarperCollins team enough for backing a second book. Every day I think how lucky I am to be working with such brilliant people. And, of course, my incredible editor Caro, for dedicating so much time to putting this together and shaping the book with me, plus putting up with me constantly wanting to change how to describe all the medical cases. I'm sure by now she must be halfway there to being able to become a vet herself.

Finally, I want to thank my brother Ross, firstly because I didn't mention him in the acknowledgements of my first book, which he was pretty sore about, for his support during my final year of training, including letting me crash at his house during a work placement. Sorry! And thanks! But on a more serious note, I want to thank him for being the inspiration that sowed a seed in my mind to want to follow in his footsteps one day. In 2011, he dedicated some time to serving an impoverished community in Tanzania, and seeing how his actions changed lives, and how volunteering changed him, it made me start to contemplate whether I could use my veterinary skills one day to help people like that.

No matter how hard and tiring this profession is, I will be forever grateful that I have a skill that can change peoples' lives through helping their animals so dramatically.